PREGNANCY, OMG!

Preg·nan·cy (PREG-nuhn-see)

A combination of the Latin words for "before" (*prae*) and "be born" (*gnasci*) meaning the time in a woman's life from conception until birth.

OMG! (oh-EM-jee)

The initials of "Oh my God" (or "goodness," or even "gosh" if that better suits you). First seen in print in a letter to Winston Churchill in 1917 and used to express excitement, shock, disbelief, and many other pregnancy-related emotions.

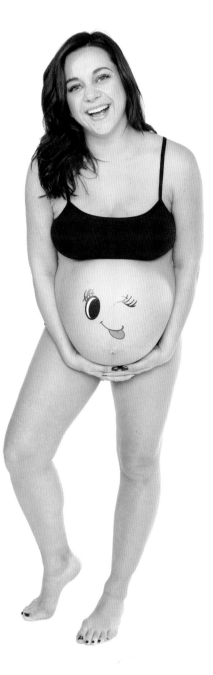

PREGNANCY, OMG!

The First-Ever PHOTOGRAPHIC Guide for Modern Mamas-to-Be

Nancy Redd

Foreword by Sherry A. Ross, MD
Photography by Brynne Zaniboni

St. Martin's Griffin
NEW YORK

Produced by Nancy Redd

www.nancyredd.com

PREGNANCY, OMG! Copyright © 2018 by Nancy Redd. All rights reserved. Printed in China. For information, address St. Martin's Press, 175 Fifth Avenue, New York, N.Y. 10010.

www.stmartins.com

The Library of Congress Cataloging-in-Publication Data is available upon request.

ISBN 978-1-250-11318-4 (trade paperback)
ISBN 978-1-250-11319-1 (ebook)

Our books may be purchased in bulk for promotional, educational, or business use. Please contact your local bookseller or the Macmillan Corporate and Premium Sales Department at 1-800-221-7945, extension 5442, or by email at MacmillanSpecialMarkets@macmillan.com.

First Edition: April 2018

10 9 8 7 6 5 4 3 2 1

This book is dedicated to my husband, Rupak, and my two children,
August and Nancy. Our little family brings me more joy than I could
have ever anticipated. I'm the luckiest mommy and wife in the world!

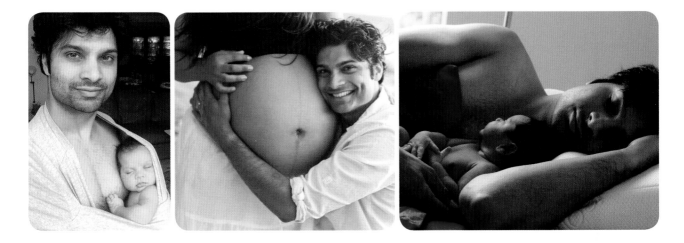

SWELLING

SKIN

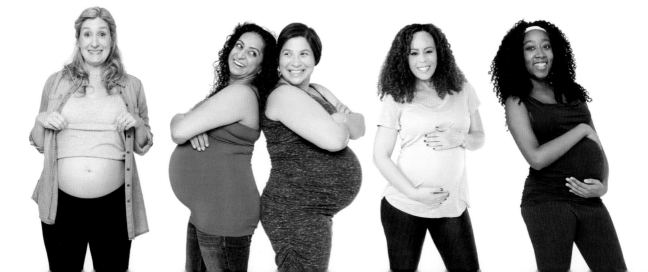

HAIR

BOOBS

DOWN THERE

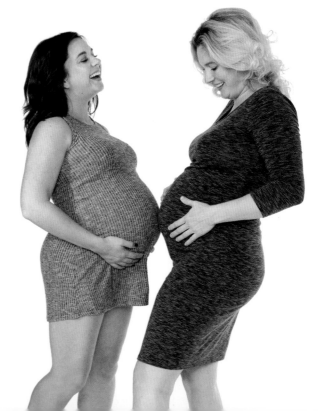

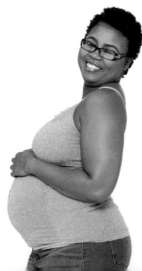

ACHES & PAINS

NOSE

EYES & EARS

HANDS & FEET

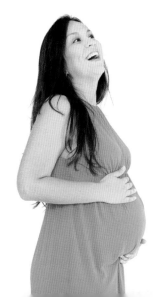

TEETH, MOUTH & THROAT

FOOD & NUTRITION

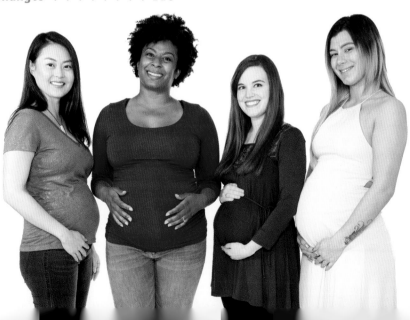

SLEEP

SEX & LOVE

MENTAL HEALTH & STRESS

NOTE FROM THE OB-GYN

As a practicing OB-GYN for the past twenty-five years, I've heard the concerns of thousands of pregnant women, not to mention having dealt with the personal challenges of my own three pregnancies. Still, I must admit: even *I* learned a few things reading this book!

I know that if ever there was a common battle cry along the pregnancy journey, it would invariably be *Oh My God!*—as in, *OMG! What's happening to my hair, voice, vagina, memory, veins, ankles?* You name it, Nancy Redd covers it in *Pregnancy, OMG!*

During pregnancy, women are especially and continuously plagued by questions concerning the changes in themselves. They go to bed with specific questions and wake up with new ones. What they crave—aside, perhaps, from foot rubs, ice cream, and potato chips (preferably all at once!)—are honest answers along with the assurance that what they're going through is at least to be expected, if not normal. Symptoms that may seem obscure in theory because only a small percent of pregnant women experience them, such as pregnancy hemangiomas (page 17) or taste distortion (page 131), in reality affect thousands of women a year who are more than just statistics. These sufferers are childbearing women who desire honest, straightforward answers and total transparency from their doctors.

Oftentimes, unfortunately, that type of unbridled frankness is hard to come by. Doctors don't always have the time for or an interest in having detailed conversations with their patients (and if they do, their answers may be too complicated and clinical for the most nimble of foggy, pregnant brains). And female friends who have been through childbirth often develop a certain amnesia about their own pregnancies (and understandably so, otherwise how many of them would go through it again?). Both of which lead to a decided (and sometimes frightening) tendency for pregnant women to rely on Dr. Google.

In my practice, as soon as an anxious yet healthy patient begins a question with, "So I Googled why I would be having vaginal spotting in the second trimester . . . ," I know I'm in for a lengthy and emotional conversation peppered with multiple reassurances on my part to set her mind at ease. In a perfect world, a patient would first come to me with her pregnancy pains and concerns instead of searching online and landing on the worst-possible-case scenario. In addition, she would have a reference that addresses her body's daily metamorphoses with equal parts integrity, insight, and humor, and a resource that illuminates all the surprising and infuriating symptoms of pregnancy she may be too embarrassed to discuss with even the closest of girlfriends. Instead, these patients are suffering and need more help than Google can offer, and that's where this book surely shines.

The particular blend of honesty and wit evident here in Nancy Redd's *Pregnancy, OMG!* is unparalleled. This is a book that answers every question you might possibly have during your pregnancy, whether it's your first or fourth. Nancy covers a host of unexpected topics, from ingrown toenails (page 98) to why women love sucking on lemons (page 131) to an embarrassing diaper rash (yours, not the baby's; page 22). Got blue lips (page 109) or have your feet grown two sizes (page 100)? Ever wondered what is meant by "lightning striking your crotch" (page 49) and "fire ears" (page 90)? You'll soon find out.

Offense is your best defense when it comes to what *really* to expect during pregnancy, and Nancy leads that offense, providing laughs and understanding every step (or pregnancy waddle) along the way.

> **Sherry A. Ross, MD**

Sheryl A. Ross, MD, "Dr. Sherry," is an award-winning OB-GYN, author, entrepreneur, and women's health expert practicing in Santa Monica, California. She is the author of *She-ology: The Definitive Guide to Women's Intimate Health. Period. The Hollywood Reporter* named Dr. Ross as one of the best doctors in Los Angeles, and Castle Connolly named her as a Top Doctor in the specialty of obstetrics and gynecology. She is also a 2017 Southern California Super Doctor.

INTRODUCTION

WHY DID NO ONE TELL ME THIS COULD HAPPEN?!

When I was pregnant with my first child, I must have ex-
claimed that exact phrase to at least a dozen mamas that I'd
known for years. The answer was almost always some version
of "We didn't want to scare you, you might not have wanted to
get pregnant." That's insanity! Knowing in advance that pregnancy might cause your voice to change (page 106) or make you
temporarily hate the love of your life's smell (page 82) isn't going to
tamp down the average woman's maternal yearning, but being prepared
for these mind and body changes can make the experience soooo much better.

I'm telling you now: You're in for one crazy ride. If this is your first pregnancy, then for
the first time in your life your body doesn't completely belong to you—you are the host to
a very cute parasite. If you've been there, done that, you're still in for a new and unusual
journey—every pregnancy is different in both beneficial and bizarre ways.

I know because I've been there, done that three times myself, and have two children to
show for it. (If you also unfortunately find yourself searching for a rainbow after suffering
a loss like I did, turn to page 186). My female friends are also all knee-deep in the fertility
years, popping out babies left and right, and we collectively became exasperated over all the
issues the other pregnancy books leave out or gloss over.

So after being a pregnant or postpartum mom for basically four nonstop years, in preparation to write this book, I scoured the Internet with fresh, nonhormonal eyes, hanging
out in popular birth-message boards, perusing blogs, and checking out what questions
preggos asked and the candid pictures they shared in the vast and anonymous online world.
I then revisited about a dozen of the top pregnancy books that caused me such angst, many
of them bearing bruised spines from being thrown across the room in terror or frustration
or both, cross-referencing them all to come up with dozens of concerns that each and every one failed to so much as acknowledge, much less advise upon. And I don't mean just a

couple of accidental misses: On the next page you will see a looong list of matters this book talks about that weren't deemed worthy of discussion by the most popular pregnancy book on the market (you know the one).

Speaking of other pregnancy books, why is it that most of 'em are organized by weeks and trimesters? Some women get hit with pregnancy nosebleeds at eight weeks and some at thirty-two. Others don't have any nausea until the third trimester, while some poor souls start getting back pain before the baby inside of them is bigger than a peanut. That's why this book is 100 percent mama-centric and organized by body part, not timetable, so you don't have to feel weird because your personal pregnancy issue is "out of order"—every pregnant body is different.

As your fingers swell up and look like sausages (page 2) and your engorged breasts seem to take on heartbeats of their own (page 38), you may feel as if your body is self-destructing. Well, stop: This book is the first ever to offer visual proof that you're not the only preggo with a purple vulva (page 50), among other disorienting dilemmas, as well as medically vetted explanations of your frustrating moments—all organized in bite-size portions designed to quickly and clearly alleviate any concerns you may have.

While I'm an expert on pregnancy *problems* (having survived zillions of my own pregnancy woes), to ensure the *advice* I give in this book is the best possible, I called on Sherry A. Ross, MD, an award-winning OB-GYN based in Santa Monica, California, and author of *She-ology: The Definitive Guide to Women's Intimate Health. Period.* She brought her invaluable first-hand experience to this book, as someone who delivers babies to hundreds of pregnant women each year, many of whom come to her practice with the same issues discussed in these pages.

This book isn't designed to give you the play-by-play of baby development, from pea to pumpkin. If you want that type of information, there are plenty of tried-and-true, fetus-focused resources, as well as your own trusted doctor, for you to turn to. Instead, this book is all about you and your body. *Pregnancy, OMG!* is here to inspire you to get through this demanding time by not only being aware of the amazing stuff that may happen to your body, but embracing rather than fearing it. Relish and rejoice in the fact that no matter what's happening to you, as you will see for yourself in this book, you are not alone!

xo, Nancy

THE DOZENS OF PREGNANCY CHANGES
THIS BOOK KNOWS YOU CAN PROBABLY EXPECT THAT
WHAT TO EXPECT DOESN'T EVEN MENTION ONCE!

Dry Mouth

Prepartum Depression

Chapped Lips

Weakened Tooth Enamel

Prenatal Mastitis

Vaginal Odor

Nose Job Changes

Pregnancy Thrush

Swollen Lips

Phantom Smells

Motion Sickness

Ulcers

Geographic Tongue

Pregnancy Hiccups

Dry Eyes

Blue Lips

Breast Implants

Tonsil Stones

Fire Ears

Pregnancy-Related Calluses

Diaper Rash (on you)

Prenatal Jewelry Allergies

Sleep Paralysis

Mouth Breathing

Excessive Sweating

Dangerous Massage Points

Watery Eyes

Loss of Smell

Gender Disappointment

Sleep Orgasms

Voice Changes

Ear Blockage

Bad Breath

Earwax Increase

Toothbrush-Induced Nausea

Taste Changes

Scent Cravings

Third Breast Growth

Ingrown Nails

Tinnitus

Cold Sores

Bunions

AND SO MUCH MORE!

SWELLING

⟫⟫⟫ If you feel like you're blowing up like a balloon, join the preggo parade! Edema is the medical term for swelling, and it affects about 80 percent of pregnant women. It also worsens throughout pregnancy. There are many reasons why we swell, some more serious than others, so read on to determine what's what.

Normal Swelling

Thanks to poor circulation coupled with a tremendous increase in bodily fluids and blood, swelling can happen in almost every nook and cranny of your body, from your face (hey, chipmunk cheeks!) to your fingers and toes.

Whether they are performed by a partner or a professional, massages are great for improving circulation and reducing swelling. Also, during the day, whenever possible, use special compression garments that are designed to put external pressure on your veins in places where you see swelling, including wrist supports or support hose for your ankles. These accessories might look and feel a bit awkward, but the pressure they apply helps alleviate pain and discomfort and reduces the risk of excess swelling and varicose veins, even in your genital area. (See page 50 for more on vulvar varicosities.)

It may seem counterintuitive, but drinking more water can help reduce swelling. Just one more reason to chug away!

Swelling That's Not Swell

No matter how absurd it might be to discover that suddenly—seemingly overnight!—your favorite tennis bracelet won't clasp because your wrist is much larger than it was pre-pregnancy, rest assured: Edema is completely normal—unless . . .

WARNING! Any of the following unusual symptoms can be a sign of a larger problem such as a heart condition, blood clot, or preeclampsia (see page 4), especially if you have a history of high blood pressure:

- **Does your swelling happen abruptly?** Sudden increases in swelling are not normal.
- **Is your swelling choosing sides?** If one leg or arm is more swollen than the other, there's something else going on.
- **Is your swelling only in your face, hands, and feet?** If the rest of your body is not swollen but these parts are, that may be a sign of preeclampsia.
- **Is your swelling accompanied by other problems?** Chest or abdominal pains, difficulty breathing, light sensitivity, intense headaches, dizziness, blurry vision, infrequent urination, and/or dysfunctional reflexes are not normal symptoms of pregnancy.

If you are experiencing any of the above issues, speak with your doctor ASAP.

> Pregnancy swelling can put you at a higher risk for a bacterial skin and/or tissue infection called cellulitis. If you have swelling paired with warmth, redness, and/or a rash, talk to your doctor ASAP as you may need an antibiotic to clear up the cellulitis before it becomes infected.

3

PREECLAMPSIA

Most sections in this book take a lighthearted look at all the weird stuff that happens to your body during pregnancy, but not this one. It's about to get dark, and necessarily so. Up to 8 percent of pregnant women suffer from a serious condition called preeclampsia, which—along with what it can evolve into, known as eclampsia—is a leading cause of death in pregnant women. Preeclampsia can restrict blood flow to the placenta, causing the baby to be underweight. It can also cause preterm birth, which may in turn involve post-delivery complications for the baby.

The exact cause of preeclampsia is not known, and any pregnant woman can develop it, though women who have high body fat or poor nutrition are believed to be at greater risk. Preeclampsia is usually seen in first pregnancies, teen pregnancies, and pregnancies among women over the age of forty. It typically is not diagnosed until after twenty weeks, but symptoms can occur much earlier, too. When you have preeclampsia and then suffer a seizure, the condition is escalated into eclampsia and is even more of a danger to you and your unborn baby.

Because many of the symptoms resemble everyday pregnancy symptoms, preeclampsia can unfortunately go unnoticed or unmentioned until it becomes a big problem, threatening the life of both mother and child. The main signs and symptoms are:

- swelling of the face, hands, and feet
- high blood pressure
- vision changes (blurry vision or seeing spots)
- abdominal pain, especially in the upper-right quadrant
- headaches
- low urine output
- shortness of breath
- sudden weight gain
- chest pain

Other risk factors for preeclampsia include:

- preeclampsia in a prior pregnancy
- pre-pregnancy high blood pressure
- obesity
- chronic medical issues such as diabetes, asthma, lupus, rheumatoid arthritis, or kidney problems
- having a first-degree relative who suffered from preeclampsia
- carrying more than one baby (a.k.a. multiple pregnancy)

If you have any of these symptoms during your pregnancy, seek medical attention right away and specifically tell your doctor your concern about possible preeclampsia.

Preeclampsia can only be alleviated by delivering the baby, but medical monitoring can improve your chances of carrying the baby to a healthy delivery date. Your doctor will almost always attempt to induce labor in a case of preeclampsia once the pregnancy is past thirty-seven weeks. If you have severe preeclampsia, you may need to deliver as soon as thirty-four weeks to ensure the safety of yourself and the baby. If the baby's lungs are not yet mature by then, your doctor may want to administer medications to promote their development, as well as medications to reduce your blood pressure, until your baby is better able to withstand delivery.

Fortunately, elevated blood pressure brought about by preeclampsia will generally lower once baby is born; however, it also increases the risk that you will have high blood pressure later in life, so try to clamp down on bad habits now to curb severe health concerns later!

⇒ Not all pain during birth is normal. Abdominal pain, especially under your ribs on your right side, should be reported to your doctor, as it is a sign of postpartum preeclampsia, especially when paired with a headache. This rare but dangerous possibility can present during labor or even a few days after childbirth, so during and after birth, make sure that your blood pressure and other vitals are being monitored just as frequently as baby's.

HOW TO ⇨ Prevent & Reduce Swelling

With these time-tested suggestions, you can aim, fire, and battle the bloat:

- **Stretch whenever you can.** Prenatal yoga, toe flexes, and other localized stretches that your doctor or physical therapist might recommend can do wonders to relieve pain and decrease swelling. Just make sure that if you are new to yoga you're sticking with poses that your increasingly unbalanced body can handle!
- **Walk and climb.** Unless your doctor orders you to limit mobility, the idea that pregnant women should refrain from physical activity is thankfully outdated. Strengthening your legs and improving your circulation through regular exercise diminishes varicose veins. Take long walks (outside or on a Stairmaster) to get your leg muscles moving, and even slowly take a flight or two of stairs (always holding on to the railing). It might leave you a little out of breath, but the health benefits are worth it.
- **Book a massage.** It feels good and gets the fluids moving. But see the massage cautions on page 76.
- **Move around often.** Try not to stay in the same position for long periods of time. If you usually stand up, make sure to take regular breaks to sit down. If you have a sitting job, get up to walk around periodically.
- **Wear comfortable shoes.** I cannot say this enough! Bedazzle your sneakers if you need to be fancy.
- **Don't cross your legs (as if you could, anyway!).** This can interfere with blood flow in your legs, increasing the risk of both varicose veins and spider veins.
- **Keep your legs up.** When sitting or lying, raise your legs above the level of your heart to speed up circulation to your legs. A pillow between the box spring and mattress near the foot of the bed helps to unobtrusively elevate your legs during sleep.
- **Sleep on your left side.** This improves blood flow from the legs back to the heart by reducing the pressure on the vena cava, a large vein on the right side of your body.
- **Limit salt intake.** Although there is no scientifically established correlation between salt intake and swelling, anecdotal evidence suggests that switching from potato chips to baked potatoes (and other whole foods) seems to help. Regardless, lowering the amount of sodium you get from prepackaged foods can only have a positive impact on your pregnancy and health.

SKIN

>>> We all know what a beautiful experience it can and should be to bring a new life into the world, but sometimes your skin doesn't get the memo. Instead, your skin, which is after all your body's largest organ, tends to be extra-sensitive during pregnancy for reasons that are not always clear. Learn how to get a handle on your hormone-rattled hide—and why it looks the way it does—on the following pages.

Hyperpigmentation

Your rising estrogen levels are increasing your melanin production, so you may, like most pregnant women, develop areas of hyperpigmentation—whether it's the darkening of pre-existing freckles, moles, or scars, a deeper nipple hue, or a condition called linea nigra (see page 9). Hyperpigmentation can occur anywhere on your body during pregnancy, including your armpits and genitals.

Skin discoloration doesn't affect the health of you or your baby, though it can drive you crazy if it catches you by surprise, as it did for me. I thought my armpits were just weirdly dirtier, and I'd scrub myself raw in the shower, until I finally complained to my doctor, who explained what was really going on.

Most treatments for hyperpigmentation are useless—and can cause more harm than good for you and baby—during pregnancy. Fortunately, the discoloration often goes away after birth.

Hyperpigmentation should not cause pain or discomfort, so tell your doctor if you notice any accompanying itchiness or tenderness, as these could be signs of another medical issue.

Linea Nigra

Before pregnancy, you had an invisible or barely perceptible pale line down the center of your stomach called the linea alba ("white line" in Latin). Most women find that in pregnancy this line widens and darkens, extending all the way from the rib cage to the pelvic bone—and for unknown reasons.

Cast your negativity aside: Some Eastern cultures view this vertical line as part of the body's "conception vessel" for purposes of reflexology and acupuncture. Consequently, the darkened linea nigra is believed to be a positive expression of an intense concentration of life-affirming energy, called chi.

Most women find that their linea nigra fades and goes away on its own before baby's first birthday. If yours doesn't and you are nursing, steer clear of bleaching creams, as many contain chemicals that might be harmful to baby. Some women find that rubbing lemon juice on the line lightens it, while others report that their lines eventually disappeared in a few years.

Pregnancy Glow

That enviable pregnancy glow is not just a myth (or a mirage). It's the result of an increase in estrogen production (particularly the estriol form), which ramps up collagen production and creates a smoother, dewier, softer, and younger skin appearance and texture in many fortunate pregnant women.

Scientists are trying to capture this pregnancy-glow phenomenon (a.k.a. fountain-of-youth miracle!) for use in antiaging skin treatments, and you may need this help sooner than you might expect. One of the reasons new moms go from luminous to lackluster in the first few postpartum months is that lack of sleep negatively affects facial collagen, creating a more haggard appearance. And no one is more sleep-deprived than a new mommy right after baby is born!

Skin Tag: You're It!

Small pieces of dangling skin called skin tags often crop up during pregnancy, especially in the second half. Though they don't hurt or itch, these little fleshy bits—typically the same shade or slightly darker than your normal skin color—are still unwelcome additions. Skin tags can show up on your neck and eyelids, beneath your breasts, in your armpits, on your stomach, and even in your groin or around your genitals.

Steer clear of medicines designed for removal, as the chemicals might not be safe for your baby. Other methods of removal done incorrectly can lead to infection and scarring, so don't attempt them at home. Besides, these harmless growths often disappear after you give birth, and you can see a dermatologist to have them safely snipped off if they don't.

Stretch Marks

Stretch marks in pregnancy are also referred to as striae gravidarum, if you want to get technical about it. They usually appear on the abdomen, where the uterus stretches the skin, but they can also crop up on your thighs, breasts, buttocks, and arms—usually as red or purple, and often itchy, streaks that can be very wide or very thin.

While stretch marks will eventually fade somewhat (emphasis on *somewhat*), they will almost always mark you for life as a mother—so sport them with pride. They're an equal-opportunity offender, too: Most pregnant women end up with at least some of these mom-markers, regardless of their age, race, and general health, and even how much weight they gained during pregnancy (a common misbelief).

It is near impossible to determine whether you're going to win or lose the "body-line lottery" until you push

> *Do pregnant women tend to get more stretch marks on one side than the other? Why yes: the outside!*

that baby out. Don't waste your money on expensive creams—they may relieve the itch and improve the appearance of stretch marks temporarily, but their long-term effects are minimal or nonexistent. Instead, soothe and hydrate your body with natural products such as coconut oil that will help relieve the itch for a fraction of the cost, and without any burning sensations; coconut oil will also help to prevent infection in case of broken skin, for a triple-win solution.

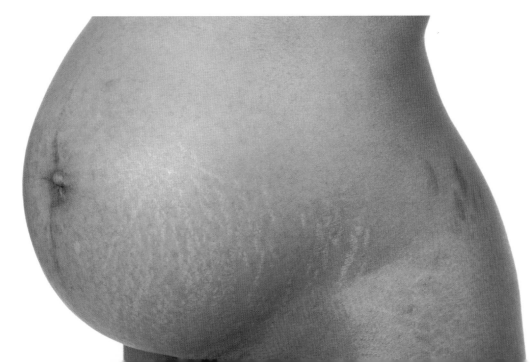

Stretching Tattoos

A growing baby is exciting, sure, but it can also spell disaster. After birth, you can look forward to poop on your expensive jeans and vomit on your favorite shirt. Even before birth, your baby can ruin some of your favorite features: your tattoos. Because your abdomen and breasts expand the most during pregnancy, tattoos in these areas often end up distorted or even split right through with a stretch mark or two—so you'll want to avoid getting a new tat in these susceptible spots while you're pregnant. After your pregnancy, you can always get a cover-up tattoo in honor of the baby who may have messed up the first one!

If you're tatted above your tushy and want pain management during delivery, never fear: There's no truth to the legend that lower-back tattoos make epidurals impossible!

Popped-out Belly Button

A popped-out belly button happens when your uterus expands and your abdomen is pushed forward, taking your navel with it. Your belly button, or umbilicus, is the remnant of your own umbilical cord that was cut when you were born—some belly buttons go in after they heal, and some go out, appearing as a little bump. If your pregnancy pops your belly button way out and you find it chafing on your clothes, medical tape is a safe and painless way to keep your navel covered and friction free. After delivery, your uterus will shrink, and most of the time your belly button will go back to its former innie or outie self.

In rare cases, your belly button can stick out so much during pregnancy that it becomes an umbilical hernia, which results when pressure from an internal organ (probably displaced by the baby) causes your abdominal muscles to tear or stretch. While this is painful for some, it usually poses no problem (other than looking weird), and your doctor will be able to keep an eye on it to ensure it doesn't lead to serious complications.

If you think your belly button is relocating, you're not imagining things. Displacement of the umbilicus, as it is formally called, usually happens toward the right side and sticks around until the abs eventually bounce back in the postpartum months. Many preggos also experience a tingling sensation around their belly button as their uterus expands—a phenomenon that also resolves after giving birth.

Pregnancy Acne

While a lucky 50 percent of mamas-to-be get that gorgeous pregnancy glow (see page 10), the other half end up with stressed-out skin. Pregnancy acne ranges from a few craters to a full-blown face freak-out, but it is almost always a temporary problem. Instead of racing to the drugstore to buy medication that might be harmful to baby (see below), embrace your inner teenager when it comes to your skin care routine:

- **Use products designed for sensitive skin.** Now is not the best time to start breaking out the antiaging creams with billions of ingredients.
- **Avoid oily or alcohol-based products.** Skin and hair products that contain oil just add fuel to the fire. On the flip side, alcohol-based products can cause dryness, which tends to ramp up oil production.
- **Wash your face twice daily.** Gently scrub your skin with a cotton pad or clean washcloth dampened with lukewarm (not hot) water. Do this morning and night, and no more; cleaning your skin too often can cause an increase in the skin's oil production.
- **Change your pillowcases regularly.** Sleeping with bacteria buildup (ewww!) doesn't help acne, so replace your cases often. This way they'll also be free of pregnancy drool, a whole other issue (see page 104).
- **Don't touch or pop your pimples!** Pregnancy acne is usually temporary, but pregnancy acne scars can be permanent.

No matter how terrible your skin starts to look, common skin-saving meds such as Accutane (isotretinoin) and related topicals, including Differin (adapalene), Tazorac (tazarotene), and Retin-A (tretinoin), can cause birth defects and other problems—as can oral hormone medications. Even tetracycline and other antibiotics used to treat acne are proven to discolor baby teeth in utero, so steer clear of these, too.

As hard as it may be to hear, you'll need to wait until after giving birth before searching for a medical solution. Even then, it may take some time for your skin to settle down again. Be prepared to experiment with different products to see which ones do the trick.

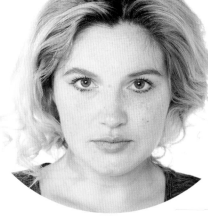

Pregnancy Mask

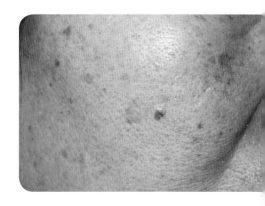

Does it look like you have a permanent chocolate milk mustache or someone smeared a bit of mud on your cheeks? Melasma gravidarum, also known as "the mask of pregnancy," is a skin condition involving discoloration that resembles splatters, dirty patches, and blotches and shows up mostly on the face—specifically the cheeks, forehead, upper lip, and chin.

Genetics and ethnicity play a huge role in who ends up resembling a Jackson Pollock knock-off. In one survey, nearly half of pregnant Pakistani women developed melasma versus only 5 percent of French women. Other studies show that women with dark hair are more prone to melasma than those with lighter shades, a finding that's in keeping with the widespread belief that women with more melanized skin types, such as African Americans and Latinas, are predisposed to developing the condition.

Pregnancy mask usually fades in the postpartum phase, and you can lower your risk of having it altogether by limiting your sun exposure. However, if staying out of the sun isn't a viable (or desirable) option, always apply a quality sunscreen, preferably one that's boosted with zinc oxide, before venturing outside. One study found that melasma cases decreased from 50 percent to 3 percent when women used sunscreen with an SPF rating of 50 or higher—and that's the smart solution for you, too.

Erythema Nodosum

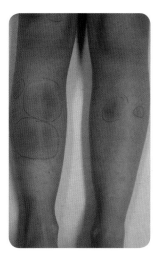

About 5 percent of pregnant women develop raised, sore nodules that can change color from red to purple to brown, as if your skin were bruised. This condition occurs mostly on your shins, though it can also appear elsewhere. Erythema nodosum is usually harmless (though sometimes painful), sporadic (it can come and go throughout pregnancy), and temporary (usually disappearing after giving birth). If the discomfort is unbearable, your doctor can prescribe a steroid cream after diagnosis.

Spider Veins

Those thin red, blue, or purple lines that are starting to creep slowly around the surface of your skin are usually called spider veins, or thread veins. They can commonly appear in many places on your body during pregnancy, most often on your neck, face, arms, upper chest, and legs. Your genes often determine whether you'll get spider veins, and unfortunately, they tend to multiply with each pregnancy. They're smaller than, but similar to, varicose veins (see below), another pregnancy side effect. Unlike varicose veins, spider veins are almost always painless, though they can be painful to look at.

For spider veins located on your legs, wearing compression stockings (and trying the other tips for swelling on page 6) might help somewhat by keeping the blood flowing more smoothly through your veins. Other than that, there's nothing you can do about most spider veins except wait it out—they usually go away after giving birth.

Varicose Veins

Over 70 percent of pregnant women deal with varicose veins, which happen when your previously normal veins become swollen and dilated thanks to a sluggish circulation system. There's no way to sugarcoat it: Varicose veins look terrible and can cause discomfort and

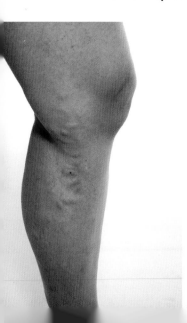

sometimes pain. While they appear most often in the legs, varicose veins can also occur in the genital area. (See the *Down There* section that starts on page 47 for information on genital varicosities such as hemorrhoids and vulvar varicose veins.)

As with spider veins (see above), which you can develop at the same time, varicose veins can worsen with each pregnancy. If you're vain about your veins, you can hide them with makeup, but regardless, they tend to decrease or vanish after giving birth—especially if you address the symptoms now by using compression garments and following the other tips for swelling on page 6.

Hemangiomas

When babies get hemangiomas—birthmarklike tumors that are visible on or just beneath the skin—we call them "strawberry kisses." But they can pop up on pregnant women, too, especially in the second trimester, when extra estrogen causes blood vessels and capillaries to multiply and become tangled.

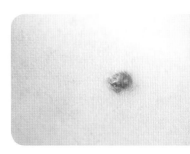

Common areas where you might develop a hemangioma include your neck and face, and they can be as small as a freckle or as big as a nipple; they can also feel flat or raised and tend to bleed easily. Even though you may want to banish these unsightly spots right away, your doctor will more than likely advise waiting until after delivery to do so.

Excess Sweat

Hyperhidrosis, or excessive sweating, doesn't come about in pregnancy because of anything you are eating or otherwise doing. It's just par for the course thanks to your elevated body temperature and ramped-up sweat glands. Hyperhidrosis often comes on strongest at night—nothing like waking up drenched in sweat to make for a perfect pregnancy! This, too, shall pass once baby is here. Interestingly, though your body may be a soggy mess, studies show your palms won't be as sweaty. Be thankful for small blessings!

Hot Flashes

Hot flashes don't just strike during menopause: About half of pregnant women suffer from unexpected bouts of facial flushing, profuse sweating, and feeling like their body has suddenly morphed into a microwave oven. Sure, older mothers closer to the onset of menopause are more likely to experience hot flashes, but women of any age can suffer from this pregnancy symptom. Hot flashes in pregnancy may be embarrassing and uncomfortable, but they aren't dangerous to you or your baby, and they don't require any special medical intervention. Sipping on plenty of ice water can cool you down a bit and may be helpful in dealing with the symptoms.

To prevent hot flashes, get up and go: Studies show that pregnant women who engage in some form of exercise have fewer symptoms—perhaps because it helps to reduce stress, thought to be an aggravating factor. Eating protein-packed meals every three to four hours also helps, as does skipping dessert—refined carbohydrates found in sugary sweets can increase your hot-flash risk. Some studies find acupuncture to be helpful with warding off hot flashes, too—as well as being an effective de-stressor.

Excess Itchiness

Itching in pregnancy is extremely common—and unbelievably annoying. Most pregnant women will simply have the occasional itch, especially in the steadily stretching belly area, but one in five is likely to experience such severe itching that it interferes with daily activities and, even worse, with sleeping. In this condition, known by the highfalutin name of pruritus of pregnancy, the itching is related to the pregnancy itself, and it tends to affect the whole body (not just the abdomen). Pruritus of pregnancy has several causes, detailed on the next few pages.

Most types of itches can be eased by adding baking soda or colloidal oatmeal to your bathwater. Slathering your skin frequently with a soothing lotion can also help—be sure to look for products that are hypoallergenic, so you're relieving rather than aggravating the irritation!

If your itching is out of control, don't run to the drugstore for DIY relief. Instead, call your doctor, who may prescribe antihistamines or oral corticosteroids such as prednisone. She may also suggest an over-the-counter corticosteroid medication such as 10 percent hydrocortisone cream.

Ignore your itch instincts and rub, don't scratch! Scratching itchy spots with your fingernails can cause even more damage to your skin and exacerbate the irritation. Vigorous rubbing with a warm, damp washcloth is safer and more effective at relieving the itch. Applying a moisturizing oil, such as coconut oil, will also help soothe dry skin, also a source of itchiness.

Irritant Contact Dermatitis

Irritant dermatitis is quite similar to atopic eczema (see page 21), but is brought on by contact with items in your environment that may not have caused you problems pre-pregnancy, whether it's your favorite food you now have an intolerance for or allergy to (page 135), your favorite laundry detergent, or even your precious wedding ring (see page 23 for more on jewelry allergies). For irritant dermatitis, the easiest way to settle the rash is to avoid whatever is causing the irritation in the first place, which means you'll want to identify the trigger(s).

Some women report seeing improvement after following elimination diets and reducing their exposure to chemicals in detergents, soaps, and shampoos—either in place of doctor-prescribed steroids or cortisone, or when taking those medications doesn't solve the problem.

PUPPP

PUPPP, which stands for pruritic urticarial papules and plaques of pregnancy (it's also known internationally as PEP, for polymorphic eruption of pregnancy), is the most common skin disorder in pregnancy—and is basically a big itchy problem. It's not harmful to your baby, but the itchiness is very irritating to mommy (a.k.a., you!) and can even interfere with sleep. PUPPP usually starts in the abdominal area, especially around the stretch marks there, but can spread to your butt and thighs, too. The same relief for other types of itching will also work for PUPPP. Your doctor might have additional recommendations.

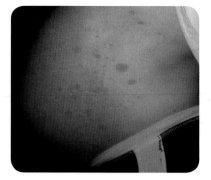

Based on studies that found a majority of PUPPP sufferers wound up delivering boys, researchers hypothesize that male fetal DNA might bring about the condition. Other possible triggers include excess weight gain in pregnancy and carrying twins, triplets, or larger-than-average babies.

Miliaria

Miliaria in pregnancy, also known as "prickly heat" or "heat rash," is caused by an increase in body temperature as well as chafing (see page 22). It looks like a pimply, red, and prickly rash (hence the nickname) and usually occurs in the folds beneath the breasts and in the groin and butt areas, and sometimes on the inside of the thighs where they rub together. Staying out of the heat and cranking up the air conditioner at home while also using the tips for treating other itchiness (see page 19) is how you'll best cope during this trying time.

Preggos with psoriasis, rejoice (at least for now)! Fifty-five percent of pregnant women who suffer from chronic psoriasis—a condition that shows up as tremendously itchy patches of scaly, thickened skin—see improvement of this autoimmune disease during pregnancy. Alas, this improvement only lasts until delivery, but don't underestimate the benefit of small favors such as these.

Pregnancy Eczema

It might seem ir-rash-ional, but many women develop some type of eczema for the first time during pregnancy, or their preexisting eczema worsens. Atopic eczema is quite common and can appear anywhere on the body as dry, itchy patches of skin that are bumpy or rough. Dyshidrotic eczema, a more severe type of eczema triggered by sweat gland activity during pregnancy, involves painful, fluid-filled blisters that can crop up on the hands and/or feet. The general treatment for eczema—moisturizers and prescription steroids—is what's used to treat eczema during pregnancy. While eczema can be annoying, even severe cases pose no harm to the baby.

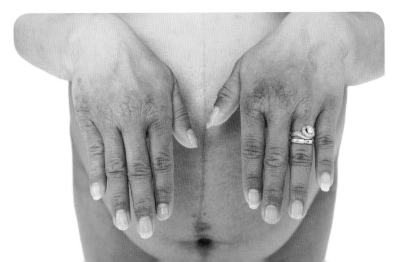

Friction and Chafing (a.k.a. "Diaper-area Rash")

Diaper rash isn't just for babies! As you gain weight, your thickening thighs often chafe due to friction created by walking. When coupled with extra moisture from additional discharge and sweat, this friction can lead to a rash in your groin and between your thighs (or your "diaper area")—a common embarrassment for many pregnant women. But chafing-related rashes can crop up anywhere on your body, including in your underarms, under your breasts, and even on your nipples.

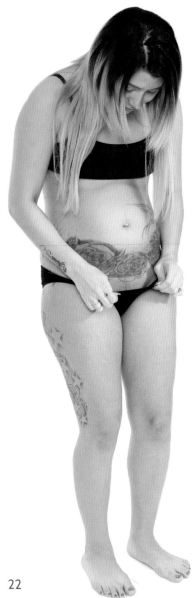

You can treat these rashes by gently cleaning the affected area and drying it completely. After you bathe and towel off, lie naked and spread-eagled across your bed. This may sound like strange advice, but following it will feel fantastic to those areas of your skin with a rash (especially your groin) and will help them heal. In cases of diaper-area rash, break out your stocked-up supply of diaper cream and talc-free baby powder and don't be ashamed to slather your sensitive parts—what works for baby's butt will safely work for yours, too. (Tidiness tip: Line your underwear with a pad to sop up excess cream and powder.)

Better yet, to help prevent chafing, wear compression clothing, such as maternity bike shorts that are knee length or longer (under your clothing!), or clothing that doesn't have a lot of seams. Wearing long skirts without underwear can also be more comfortable when you're out and about. While at home, air things out by going commando or completely naked whenever you can.

> Nipple chafing can be helped by covering your twin peaks with medical tape, which will keep your growing "girls" from rubbing against your bra. Medical tape stays put as long as you want it to—and doesn't hurt the slightest bit when it's pulled off.

Jewelry Rashes

Allergies to metals in pregnancy are not as uncommon as you may think. You yourself may suddenly find that your earlobes are itching, your ring finger has developed a rash, or your wristwatch has left behind an itchy band. If so, that's likely due to an allergy to nickel—pregnancy increases the absorption of nickel through the skin. White gold and lower-grade silver jewelry often contain nickel, but anecdotally, some women even find themselves suddenly allergic to their platinum wedding rings!

Common symptoms of metal allergies include redness, dry patches, rashes, swelling, and itching of those areas that are exposed to the metal. If you continue to wear the offending jewelry, the affected skin can thicken, become cracked and leathery, and darken. Usually these changes occur only in the area directly in contact with the jewelry, but if you have a serious metal allergy, the rash may spread to other areas of your body—it can also become infected.

Your doctor can tell whether you have an allergy to metal simply by looking at the rash and asking you questions about your exposure to jewelry, or by doing a skin patch test. While some women have found that coating the inside of their rings with clear nail polish solves the problem, this scheme does not always work. The best way to deal with a metal allergy is to avoid wearing jewelry that contains the culprit metal and to treat any rash or swelling with an OTC hydrocortisone cream (with your doctor's approval).

A jewelry allergy doesn't usually just end along with your pregnancy—once you develop the reaction, you might have it for the rest of your life, but you won't know for a few months. Not that you'll be able to wear your wedding ring for a while, thanks to probable postpartum swelling! (See page 2 for more on swelling.)

DORMANT DISEASES APPEARING IN PREGNANCY

In pregnancy, your immune system is not what it used to be. Viral diseases that normally lie dormant in your body can rear their ugly heads during this time, so be on guard.

Shingles

Some pregnant women can get herpes zoster, also known as shingles, where a section of skin becomes covered with a red, blistery, and often painful rash that looks a lot like chicken pox, and for good reason! People who contracted the chicken pox virus (or varicella-zoster virus) as a child usually still harbor the inactive virus in the nerves of the spinal cord. When those people are immunocompromised, the virus makes a comeback as shingles. Pregnancy presents just such a scenario.

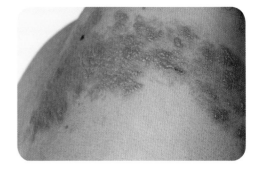

In fact, pregnant women are often tested by their doctors to see whether they are immune to the chicken pox virus. If it turns out you're not immune, your best bet is to steer clear of anyone who has an active case of chicken pox or shingles, because exposure to either form of the virus might cause you to develop chicken pox during your pregnancy, which carries risks for the baby.

That said, having an outbreak of shingles in pregnancy is usually not dangerous, but must be monitored by your doctor for possible complications such as pneumonia or encephalitis.

Genital Herpes

Nearly one in three pregnant women have herpes simplex virus (HSV), known commonly as genital herpes. If you know that you're one of them, alert your doctor now so she can plan accordingly—an outbreak during labor raises the risk of transmitting the disease to the baby. (Note: This is especially true if you contracted HSV during pregnancy; new infections pose a much higher risk of transmission and other birth complications than preexisting ones, especially if the first outbreak happens near the end of pregnancy.) Symptoms of an HSV outbreak include tingling, burning, or visible lesions.

Your doctor may recommend that you take medication during your pregnancy to prevent the virus from flaring up or, should you have an outbreak at the time of delivery, to have a cesarean section to protect your newborn from the disease.

You might not even be aware that you had herpes before becoming pregnant: About 80 percent of women with HSV infections have no symptoms—meaning that many women first discover they have genital (or other types of) herpes when their pregnancy brings on a surprise outbreak. If this happens to you, don't be ashamed. You are obviously not alone here, and you need to protect your and your baby's health by being honest with your doctor.

Try to see your doctor during an outbreak, or at least take pictures to help confirm the diagnosis. So long as no symptoms are present near your due date, vaginal delivery is usually safe despite a previously confirmed diagnosis of HSV.

Cold Sores

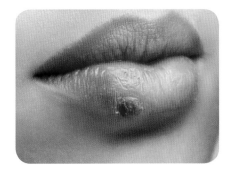

If a cold sore (or "fever blister") pops up around your lips, you, like the majority of Americans, have oral herpes. Oral herpes is not a big deal, as well over half of Americans contract it by adulthood, but you should tell your doctor as soon as an outbreak happens, especially if it's the first time you can recall having one. Cold sores are extremely common in pregnancy, thanks to an abundance of stress and hormones, and usually pose no threat to the baby.

However, if the sore is present during birth, there is the slight risk of complications, and only your doctor can determine the right course of action—including possibly prescribing a safe medication to shorten the outbreak. And if you have a case of oral herpes at delivery, you may want to hold off from kissing your newborn (and inadvertently spreading the disease) until cleared by your doctor. Oral herpes is significantly more problematic in babies than adults.

For canker sores and mouth ulcers inside of your mouth, see page 115.

Hives

Developing hives during pregnancy does not mean you're allergic to your baby (though this is a common old wives' tale). Rather (and relievedly), hives often happen because your pregnant skin is more sensitive to allergens in your environment, and because the stretched-out, drier-than-normal skin may be more prone to irritation.

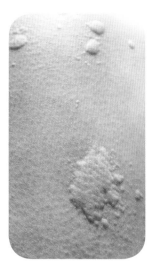

Hives are splotchy and itchy and tend to come and go, especially when you're in contact with the allergen (like a triggering fabric in your clothes) or if you are overheated. If you suffer from hives during pregnancy, your doctor can prescribe or recommend antihistamines to shrink the lesions and relieve the itching. Paying attention to what you were doing or wearing when the hives appeared is also a good idea; sometimes the cause is what you least expect—your pets, your lotion, or even your jewelry (see page 23).

Intrahepatic Cholestasis Of Pregnancy (ICP)

Your itch may need more than just a scratch; if it's ICP you may need medicine to protect the baby. Also known as obstetric cholestasis and commonly referred to as jaundice of pregnancy, ICP affects about 4 percent of pregnant women. Usually diagnosed in the third trimester (but diagnosable any time in pregnancy), this liver disease is characterized by itching (with or without the presence of bumps) and is sometimes, but not always, combined with a yellowing of the whites of the eyes and the skin (or jaundice). The itchiness is usually strongest on the palms of your hands and the soles of your feet but can spread to the rest of your body, too.

Although ICP tends to subside on its own within forty-eight hours after giving birth, you should mention any symptoms to your doctor, as this condition is often seen in combination with other problems in pregnancy. If ICP is suspected, your doctor might perform an easy diagnostic blood test and, once confirmed, may prescribe medicine to treat the bile acid buildup caused by ICP while monitoring you closely for any related issues throughout the rest of your pregnancy.

HAIR

Thicker Hair

When you're not pregnant, it's as though each hair on your head and body is wearing its own set of headphones, rocking along and taking no notice of all the other hairs nearby. This is because hair grows and hangs around for a while and then randomly falls out, only to repeat the cycle again and again. Once you're pregnant, however, you may find that most of your strands are grooving to the same beat . . . and then they all suddenly freeze, getting stuck in the growth phase.

By the second trimester, many women marvel at how thick and full their pregnancy hair seems to be. This is just an illusion: Pregnancy hair only appears thicker because all those hormones prevent many more strands from falling out compared to pre-pregnancy shedding—and especially in contrast to post-pregnancy hair loss, which is often traumatic (and leads to the classic "mom chop").

Thinning Hair & Bald Spots

On the flip side of the thicker-appearing-hair syndrome, many women find that, to their utter dismay, pregnancy comes with hair loss. This can be particularly devastating if your pre-pregnancy hair was your crowning glory and right now your crown is looking quite tarnished. I was, alas, one of these women. My hair thinned so terribly that by the middle of my pregnancy I had to wear clip-in hairpieces to look "normal" at work. Hair loss during pregnancy has many causes, including:

- pregnancy-related diabetes or anemia
- thyroid issues
- deficiencies in protein, vitamins, and minerals
- taking too much of some vitamins and minerals, including vitamin A and selenium
- certain antibiotics

Break out the mascara and brow powder, because pregnancy can cause your eyebrows and eyelashes to fall out, too.

If your hair is falling out in clumps and leaving behind noticeable bald patches, you may be one of the unfortunate women who suffer from pregnancy-related alopecia. See page 30 for a firsthand account of this unexpected side effect.

Hair Breakage

While there's nothing dull about pregnancy, the same can't always be said for your pregnancy hair. Split ends and other types of hair breakage are often more prevalent during pregnancy due to changes in the hair's texture as well as pregnancy-hormone-caused dryness, which weakens the hair shaft.

You're not the only one experiencing hair drama—your fetus is also turning into a fur baby! *Lanugo* is the term given the ultra-fine, downy hair that babies develop all over their bodies while in the womb. Most babies shed this fuzzy fleece while still in the womb, but others end up looking like an adorable little Sasquatch for a short while after birth. (Trust me: It always goes away.)

⮕ TRUE STORY:

PREGNANCY MADE ME BALD!

BY MOLLY ERDMAN

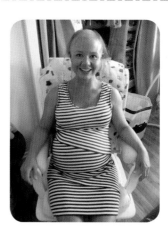

Six months into my pregnancy, I gave myself a hearty pat on the back for how great I was handling everything. Sure, there had been some discomfort here and there, but all that was behind me. I was nailing it! Those were a fun couple of days. Then my scalp started itching. Three months later, I would be completely bald.

Soon after the itching started, I noticed more than the usual hair in my brush and on the bathroom floor. And on my pillow. And on every other surface in our home. I started combing my hair directly over the trash can, watching a toupee-worthy number of strands cascade down. I scoured the Internet for answers. There were countless stories of women losing hair after giving birth, but none about losing hair during pregnancy. My doctor simply chalked it up to "one of those things!" Oh, pregnancy! Seriously, though–that was his answer. Soon my hair was coming out in fistfuls. I never left home without a hat or bandana because my bare scalp was visible in several spots.

One morning my mom called, urging me to have my thyroid checked. She and my grandmother had both experienced low thyroid levels, and she wondered if that might explain my hair loss. Being over thirty-five, I had already had my thyroid checked in the buffet of tests early in my pregnancy, but I convinced my doctor to test it again. Mom was right: My thyroid hormone level was low. I started on Levothyroxine, but my doctor warned me my follicles had likely already shut down and the hair-loss cycle would have to finish before regrowth could begin. He offered something glib about how most "wacko" things that happen during pregnancy magically return to normal after delivery.

I spent much of my remaining pregnancy feeling pretty weepy. With a month to go, my hair had become what my husband described as "Gollum-esque," which would seem cruel if he weren't such a huge *Lord of the Rings* fan. On my due date, my doctor informed me I was nowhere near going into labor, and I burst into tears. I could not wait to meet this baby girl, whom I assumed would be born with a full head of hair in some weird circle-of-life thing. I wanted this pregnancy to be over, and I needed to know if my hair was coming back.

Twelve days later Valerie was born, and I instantly forgot I was bald. Soon, stubble started to burst forth, and within a few months I myself had a full head of short, mom-practical hair–and a story that can trump almost any round of It Happened to Me.

Chemical-free Hair Care

Of course, you always want to look your baby mama best, but now is not the time to put vanity before valor. It is the time, however, to carefully read the labels on the stuff you slather on your scalp and to consider which products you should squirrel away for the next few months. While most of the research suggests that chemical processes such as hair dyeing or straightening pose little risk to the fetus, a handful of smaller studies haven't been so certain in their findings.

One problem mamas-to-be run into is this: If your scalp has a current abscess, burn, or open sore (from, say, scratching your head), anything that comes into contact with that area of your scalp can take a bullet train (i.e., the blood coursing through your veins) directly to your placenta. In most cases, your body breaks down the chemicals before they can do any harm, but an open wound gives chemicals carte blanche to enter your bloodstream.

Because you might not be aware of tiny cuts or sores on your scalp, it's almost impossible to know whether you're in the clear to use products with chemicals. As such, your best bet is to:

- **Forgo single-process hair dyes altogether.** You'll save so much money and have such peace of mind! Bust out your old headbands and touch up your roots for as long as you can with specialty mascara-wand applicators or brush-on powders sold in most beauty-supply stores. An alternative is to opt for highlights and lowlights that are painted onto your hair rather than applied to your scalp.
- **Also forgo relaxers or other chemical straighteners.** There just hasn't been enough research to establish the safety of the chemicals used in either lye or no-lye relaxers. Better to be safe (and curly!) than sorry.
- **Reconsider your products.** Remember that during pregnancy your hair color, texture, and growth may change. Hair products that you used before pregnancy might interact differently with your hair now.

If you do decide to use chemical products, be sure to take the following precautions:

- **First do a patch test on your forearm.** Now that you're pregnant, you could have a sensitivity or allergic reaction to products you've used for years.
- **Look for scalp wounds.** Make sure that you have no sores, scratches, or open abscesses on your scalp. This may require your partner to do a deep dive on your behalf, parting your hair multiple times to get a good look at your scalp. If any wounds are found, don't take the risk.
- **Avoid noxious odors.** Take steps to avoid breathing in chemical fumes emitted from any hair processes you undertake at home (or at the salon). Make sure the space you're in is well ventilated; better yet, wear a mask (or do both to be on the super-safe side).
- **Wear gloves.** Always protect your hands when using dyes or other strong chemical-based products (whether you are pregnant or not).

My hat is off to you if you can hold off on chemical hair processes until your baby's born. Or perhaps, in this case, I should say, "Hats on!"

Oily Hair

If your scalp is overproducing sebum and your hair is limp and slick and greasy looking, you are not alone. Switching to a new shampoo and conditioner for oily hair, as well as using dry shampoo between washings, often helps to ride out the oily tidal wave.

Texture & Color Changes

Your hair might also decide to throw you a curveball by changing its pattern of growth. If it's normally fine and straight, you might start seeing some coarseness or wave action, or vice versa (see the True Story on page 33). Even if you don't color your hair, you could see a line of demarcation as your pregnancy hair—above the line—might be darker than your pre-pregnancy hair.

TRUE STORY:
PREGNANCY MADE ME LOSE MY CURLS!

BY COURTNEY M. WILLIAMS

When I was little, I had straight hair. When I entered the earliest stages of puberty, around third grade or so, my hair became super-curly and stayed that way until I had my first child.

As my postpartum hair fell out in clumps, I decided to chop it off and get a "mom cut." It was while looking in the mirror after that haircut that it dawned on me: My hair wasn't curly anymore! My pre-pregnancy corkscrew spirals lay on the salon floor and I was left with merely wavy hair, all seemingly in the blink of a sleep-deprived eye.

I suddenly had a flashback to when I was getting a haircut in college, and the stylist warned me that I'd lose my curls when I got pregnant. I'd blown him off at the time, but now here I was, and he turned out to be right. It sounds crazy, but since pregnancy had certainly altered my shoe size, it wasn't such a stretch to think that yes, pregnancy made me lose my curls.

A coworker of mine witnessed her hair go from stick straight to very curly with her first pregnancy, and from very curly to wavy with her second. So for a while I held out hope that my hair might change back with my second pregnancy. Alas, it wasn't meant to be. My first child is six years old and my second is almost four, and my hair remains merely (albeit manageably) wavy. I still miss my signature curls, but I've made peace with my new do.

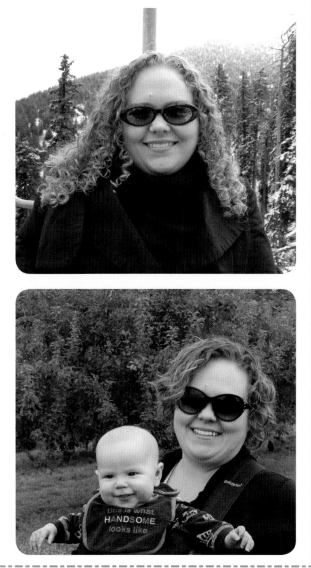

Excess Body Hair

Because your hormones are throttling in overdrive, you might see more hair blooming on your arms and legs than on a baby chimp, and inexplicable strands sprouting on your face, belly, and even your boobs. Just another rest stop on the rocky road of pregnancy indignities. It might feel like a losing battle, but you do have a few options in trying to combat the dreaded hair flare-up:

- **DIY only the parts that you can see.** For facial, nipple, and belly hair, tweezing and threading are the best options for now, as the verdict is still out on the safety of bleaching and depilatory creams.
- **Enlist help with the rest.** Don't try to tackle the hair on parts of your body that you can no longer reach. You've dispatched your partner on midnight runs to fulfill your food cravings and requested help in remembering times and dates when "pregnancy brain" gets the best of you, so it's no biggie to ask him to help you shave your legs, too.
- **Better yet, let a professional handle everything.** That's why salons and spas were invented, right? When you're pregnant, you deserve pampering. A quiet room and time spent with your favorite esthetician is as close to bliss as it comes.
- **Give up!** Get in touch with your inner hippie or ancestral cavewoman. Make friends with your new coat of hair. Once your baby is born, shaving won't be near the top of your wish list for some time. Might as well get used to being a little fuzzy right now.

Here are a few other things you should keep in mind when feeling the urge to purge (your body hair, that is):

- **Never, ever try to shave your legs while standing in the shower.** Your baby bump has shifted your center of gravity, making it easy for you to lose your balance and fall. Instead, sit on the edge of the tub with your feet on the floor (not in the tub, as that's more dangerous). If you're going electric, you can sit wherever you're most comfortable, including on a sturdy bench or the edge of the bed.

- **Don't shave what you can't see.** You might be—literally—itching to shave your coochie, but don't do it if you can't see it. Nicks and cuts in your nether region can easily get infected, and shaving down there when you can't see what you're doing is a job best reserved for your partner or a paid professional who can steer clear of your sensitive bits (ouch!).

- **Do a patch test when waxing or sugaring.** Just like a zillion other body weirdnesses that crop up during pregnancy, your skin sensitivity changes. Whether it's your bikini area, legs, face, or another body part, doing a quick test before slathering your skin in goo will prevent a situation where a little hair is the least of your worries. The same goes whether you are at home or in a salon; the technician can do a quick patch test on your arm to make sure you're good to go.

- **Weigh the risks carefully.** While electrolysis is an absolute no-go in pregnancy, laser hair-removal treatments seem to be technically safe but can cause permanent scarring and changes in pigmentation. It's always a good idea to check with your doctor and follow her recommendations when it comes to permanent hair removal. And remember: Your new fur is probably temporary, making it even less worth any potential side effects.

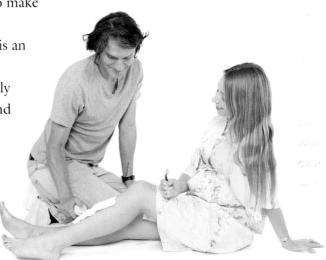

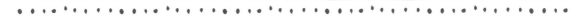

Are you an ardent fan of laser hair removal? Don't be surprised if all the money you spent pre-pregnancy goes down the drain — pregnancy often permanently restimulates hair follicles, promoting new hair growth.

Waxing Before Labor

While there are pros and cons to having a prebirth wax, one point isn't in dispute: Doctors and nurses could not care less whether your quim is hairy or sleek. They've seen it all—and then some.

The two main arguments against waxing soon before delivering are that it can be expensive to have it done in a good salon (and you should only ever get waxed in a good salon) and, if you've never been waxed before, you may find it rather painful.

The argument in favor of waxing is mostly cosmetic. If you're self-conscious about your pubes and you believe a good Brazilian wax will instill the confidence you'll need in the delivery room, go for it. (Chances are, though, that once you're in the throes of labor, you'll give exactly zero figs about your pube-do.)

A strong case can also be made for prebirth waxing based on hygienic grounds: The lack of hair down there can help in caring for stitches (if any) and with cleaning off clotted blood, of which there will be lots if you have a vaginal delivery.

If you are going to wax, do it right. Choose a salon or spa that's sparkly clean. Your esthetician should always wear gloves and use a new spatula (if not, ewww!), and there absolutely must not be any double dipping (double ewww!). Either she should start with a small pot of wax that is just for you, or, if not (triple ewww!), she should use a new stick every time she dips into the wax. An antiseptic lotion on your hoo-ha before and after your wax will also help avoid infection—and soothe any irritated skin.

An alternative to a bikini wax is a bikini shave, but if you're planning on removing your pubes, go for the wax to avoid feeling itchy after delivery. As you heal you are not going to be able to shave, nor will you even want to—that's guaranteed.

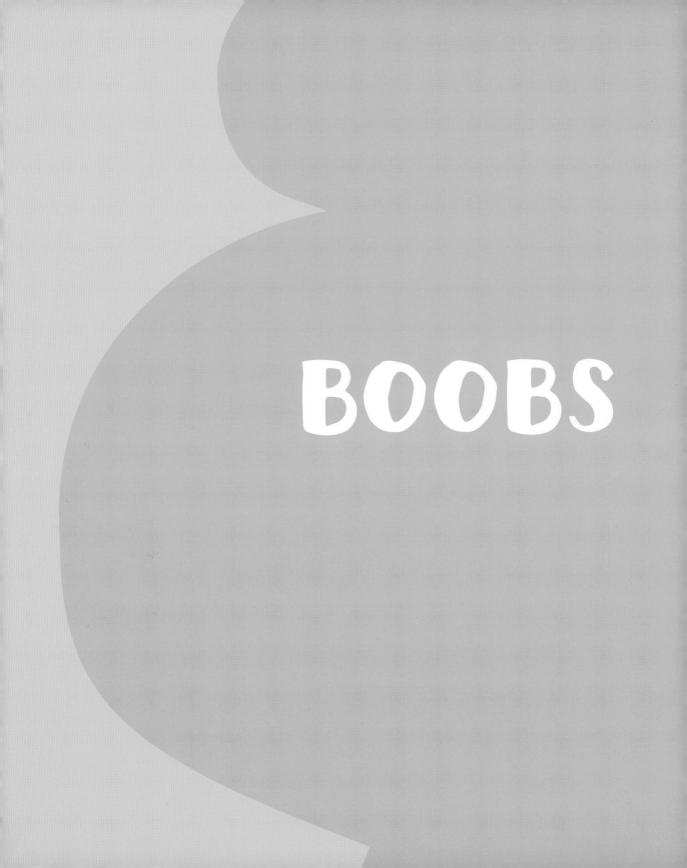

BOOBS

> Now that you're pregnant, it may seem as if your body is treating your breasts to a massive remodeling project, upgrading them from sensuous body parts to functional food machines in just a few months. It's all too true! Read on to learn about the titillating changes happening to your breast friends.

Painful Breasts

As the surrounding skin stretches and your internal breast structure rapidly develops the capacity for milk secretion, the physical responses of soreness, tenderness, tingling, heaviness, and even itching (oh my!) are completely normal, albeit frustrating. Soothing your traumatized ta-tas with cold compresses (see page 39) can help to ease the pain.

Sometimes, however, your boobs might malfunction as they transform into milk makers. Signs that your breast pain may be more than mere growing pains include:

- redness, rash, or other types of inflammation
- pus or discharge from anywhere on the breast or nipple
- isolated lumps
- intense pain or burning
- any of the above, accompanied by low-grade fever, rash, chills, or aches

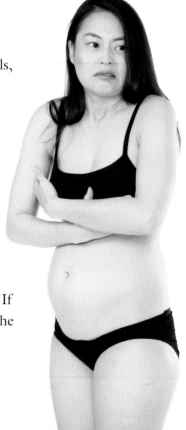

Possible explanations for your more-than-normal breast pain include a bacterial infection or even nonlactational mastitis. While mastitis is mostly a problem for women who are breastfeeding, it sometimes plagues women in pregnancy as well. Any trauma to the breast, like an accidental punch or a bump into a wall, can also shake things up in a not-so-great way.

If you feel that your breast pain is other than general, talk to your doctor. If she brushes you off, listen to your maternal instinct and keep persisting until you find someone who will listen. If there truly is an issue, the longer you wait without intervention, the more painful and problematic it will likely become.

Bra Talk

Don't waste money on multiple bras during pregnancy, because your cup size is constantly changing! Instead, pick up a bra extender, which will only set you back a couple of dollars—the extra band width will buy you a few extra months' time. On

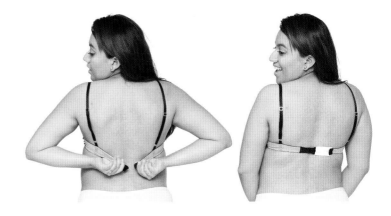

casual days, a front-zip sports bra not only will feel comfortable on your growing chest, but also will be useful in the postpartum months—bonus points if the bra's band and shoulder straps are adjustable.

If you do treat your bosom buddies to a new bra, look for one that gives them the support they need while also limiting any pain from chafing or movement, and without crushing their essential milk ducts (hint: no underwire).

HOW TO ▷ Make Cold Compresses For Breast Pain

Those bags of frozen peas tucked away in your icebox are more than a convenient way to get your daily fill of veggies—they're also handy ice packs for soothing breast pain, and much more formfitting than standard packs. When your breasts start to hurt, lie down with a towel covering your chest (to help avoid freezer burn) and press two bags of frozen vegetables (one for each boob) on top of the towel. You can do this for other bodily aches and pains, too—pregnant or not.

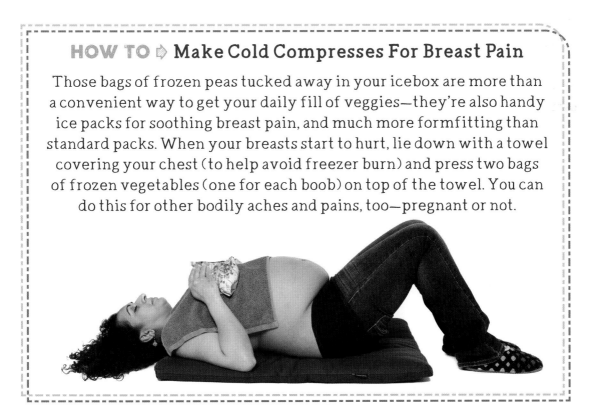

Nipples From (o)(o) To (@)(@)

Being squeezed out of a vagina can certainly work up an appetite, but brand-new babies can't even find their own thumbs to suck, let alone another person's boob. That's why nature compels your nipples and areolas to deepen in color and increase dramatically in size: The bigger and darker the targets, the easier it will be for your baby to find them. Just think how calves and other baby mammals can easily find their mommas' udders to latch on to. We humans are admittedly a bit more evolved—and thankfully, our "udders" don't grow (or sag!) nearly as much as Bessie's. But you get the picture.

Because biology does not prioritize (or even acknowledge) our human vanity, this new pigmentation will often be uneven, and it may also resemble a bull's-eye as your secondary areola expands in circumference, surrounded by a lighter, irregular ring that may, or may not, darken over time.

While your darker, larger areolas may fade and/or partially shrink, they will almost never return to their exact pre-baby size and coloring—and that's OK! Consider it the new normal.

See-through Skin

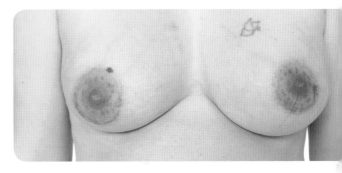

Because the skin around your breasts is stretching so quickly, you might suffer some physical discomfort such as itching. At times, the skin may also appear paper-thin or even completely transparent, meaning all those vascular patterns that were previously invisible to the naked eye can now be seen in their full glory—no ultrasounds or x-rays needed!

What's more, the many veins crisscrossing your breasts and nipples appear darker than elsewhere because the body is pumping an increased blood supply to this area. If you find all of this unsettling, join the club—and remember that it's for a good reason (your baby's nourishment).

Bumpy Nipples

You'll likely notice many small, protruding bumps popping up around the nipples and on the nipples themselves. Some of these bumps connect to your milk ducts, but others are dilated sebaceous glands called Montgomery's tubercles, which have always been there (who knew?) but now have a bit more work to do. If you're planning on breastfeeding, these tiny glands are your new best buds. The oily substance they produce, known as lipoid fluid, is a natural lubricant that protects the nipples against cracking from baby's near-constant feeding (consider yourself forewarned!).

Interestingly, several research studies show that this fluid also acts like an olfactory stimulant for babies—the smell gets them pumped up for breastfeeding and offers a way for your own newborn to recognize and call dibs on your breast milk as hers for the taking. Good news: Your so-called boob wax will cease production shortly after you stop nursing.

Female humans are the only mammals to develop full breasts and prominent nipples regardless of lactation. Other mammals—from pigs to platypuses— only have this honor when they are pregnant with or nursing their babies.

Leaky Nipples

If your nipples start to leak weeks, or even months, before your due date, it's nothing to fret about. This clear (or yellowish) sticky liquid, which forms a crust when it dries on your skin or clothes, is called colostrum. It differs from milk in color, consistency, taste, and composition, and is crucial to supporting the health of your baby.

Colostrum has a unique makeup that's easier for newborns to digest, while also being nature's most perfectly balanced food, containing high amounts of proteins and vitamins as well as human growth factors. In fact, if you catch a cold, your boobies will know, and they'll create antibodies to pass along to your baby. A little doubtful? One study found that colostrum cells produced antibodies rapidly after being exposed to a nonpathogenic strain of *E. coli*.

> Some women report having leaky breasts, typically only in small amounts, for years after their babies are born.

Colostrum also facilitates your baby's first poop, medically referred to as meconium; this is an important milestone because before then, nothing has passed through the rather long intestinal tract.

Every woman's body is different, though. Some moms-to-be never experience leaking before birth, while others start dripping in the first trimester. If you are leaking, the more you or your partner touches or handles your breasts, the more the leaking will persist. Unless you're leaking a discharge that is not clear or yellowish, has an unpleasant odor, or is accompanied by pain or blood, there is usually no reason to worry (but call your doctor immediately if you are leaking blood). Because you don't want to inhibit colostrum production, your only real option is to place some breast pads in your bra's cups to absorb the fluid. These pads will be useful once you begin breastfeeding, too.

Breastfeeding 101

Like women, nipples come in all shapes and sizes, and there are no defining qualities that indicate the types of nipples that will provide a successful breastfeeding experience. Women with flat and inverted nipples, however, may require a little extra effort to get the milk flowing properly, so talk to your doctor in advance and don't take no for an answer. As a card-carrying flat-nippled breastfeeding mom, I am proof that anything is possible with the right support system in place.

No matter the circumstances, breastfeeding is a learned skill for both mama and baby. Although you'd think it would be instinctual, breastfeeding can require a great deal of perseverance, patience, and trial and error. Several factors help determine how smoothly breastfeeding will or won't go, such as your milk supply and your ability to find your baby's preferred feeding position.

In addition, while some babies will emerge from the womb and take to breastfeeding as though they hold a PhD in latching on, other babies will struggle to master the many mouth muscles that must work together to draw out the milk. So, regardless of what your nipples look like, take comfort in knowing that their appearance has nothing to do with whether breastfeeding will be a walk in the park or a marathon.

Implants & Breastfeeding

Some women with "perfect" natural breasts experience issues with breastfeeding. Some women with breast implants experience no issues whatsoever. Although it's an utter myth that all women with augmented boobs can never breastfeed, research does seem to suggest that at least some of them may face an uphill battle in doing so. It turns out only one-third of moms with breast implants are successful at nursing. Incision location seems to play a role—the closer it is to the underboob crease, the higher the breastfeeding success, at least according to one study.

You won't know how it will work out until you try to breastfeed yourself—so keep your fingers crossed and your eyes on the prize! There's some thinking that the reason many women with implants don't succeed at breastfeeding is that they've already psyched themselves out due to a misguided sense of stigma and shame. Don't fall prey to this negative thinking!

If you do wind up being able to breastfeed, there's another upside: Whereas natural breasts have a tendency to droop after nursing has stopped, a recent study shows that augmented breasts are likely to stay in tip-top shape. (Lucky you!)

Breast reduction procedures don't always cause breastfeeding problems, either. For some women, the resulting nerve damage does prevent them from being able to nurse their babies exclusively, but don't shy away from breastfeeding entirely— every little bit of milk you can squeeze out for your baby is beneficial, even if you must supplement it with formula.

TRUE STORY:

I GREW A THIRD, LACTATING BREAST WHILE PREGNANT

BY GENELLE BILLINGS

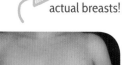

Not Genelle's actual breasts!

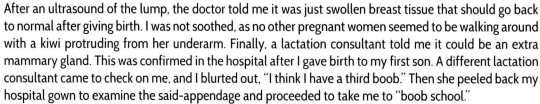

I've had five babies. My first pregnancy was the most exciting until I noticed that a kiwi-size lump was growing in my armpit. Did I have cancer? After an ultrasound of the lump, the doctor told me it was just swollen breast tissue that should go back to normal after giving birth. I was not soothed, as no other pregnant women seemed to be walking around with a kiwi protruding from her underarm. Finally, a lactation consultant told me it could be an extra mammary gland. This was confirmed in the hospital after I gave birth to my first son. A different lactation consultant came to check on me, and I blurted out, "I think I have a third boob." Then she peeled back my hospital gown to examine the said-appendage and proceeded to take me to "boob school."

Apparently, a woman's milk lines run from her armpit all the way down to her abdomen (just picture a dog nursing a litter of puppies all at once). You can be born with extra mammary glands or extra nipples anywhere along this milk line and, unless the nipple is visible, you may not know it's even there until your breasts swell during pregnancy. After this brief primer, the consultant told me about a woman with eight boobs who was in the hospital the day before. Eight. Boobs. I suddenly felt rather happy just to have the three. I was assured that my extra boob would go away after nursing, and since there was no visible nipple, the boob would dry up and shrink back to its formerly undetectable size. I nodded happily, relieved and ready to move on.

That was wishful thinking. When I first started nursing my newborn son, I felt like I was sweating profusely. When I looked down, I realized that I wasn't sweating. What I believed to be a tiny brown freckle was actually a nipple that was currently dripping milk into a puddle on my shirt. Yep—sign me up for the circus. Not only do I have a third boob, but it also lactates.

From then on, I had to nurse with a towel lodged in my armpit. While most moms just wore absorbent breast pads in their nursing bras, I got to do that *and* wear a huge Band-Aid on my armpit. Hooray for me.

Between babies one and two, I had the third boob removed surgically. There is still breast tissue in there that swells up to say "hi" with each subsequent pregnancy. But at least there isn't a nipple for the milk to leak through anymore.

So there you have it. I think my experience having a third boob can give everyone a brighter outlook on their pregnancies and after-baby bodies. Your tummy may look like a venetian blind from those hard-earned stretch marks, or you may have skin that now somehow resembles that of an elephant's trunk. Still, when looking in the mirror at yourself, you can always say, "At least it doesn't lactate." Cheers to that!

Breast Lumps

Sometimes, breast tumors will show up in pregnancy. These growths may be soft or hard, tiny or large, and are generally painless. They have many medical names, including lactating adenomas and fibroadenomas, but to you, pregnant lady, any kind of abnormal bump in your breasts is lumped together in what is thought of as Worst. Nightmare. Ever.

Do not worry! Many, if not most, tumors or lumps are benign (noncancerous), and they often existed before pregnancy and are just growing along with your baby—and boobs—in response to hormonal changes. Alert your doctor, who can ease your fears with proper testing or careful monitoring. Many growths regress on their own after the mom has given birth or after breastfeeding has ended, but keep your doctor in the loop so that she can monitor any changes.

Statues of ancient Greek and Indian goddesses sometimes have rows upon rows of breasts across their chest. Historians believe that this is because extra nipples and breasts were a prized sign of femininity and fertility.

Breast Cancer & Pregnancy

Be on the lookout for the onset of breast cancer during pregnancy, especially if it runs in your family. All in all, over one thousand American women are diagnosed with breast cancer during pregnancy each year, most of them between the ages of thirty-two and thirty-eight. In fact, up to 20 percent of breast cancers detected in women under the age of thirty years old are associated with pregnancy. That may be a scary statistic, but it doesn't have to be. It's much better to be well informed than unaware. Fortunately, to date there is no evidence indicating that breast cancer in the mother poses a threat to the baby.

Detecting lumps in the breast—the most common sign of breast cancer—can be difficult during pregnancy because, as discussed in this section, your boobs begin changing the minute your body realizes it is pregnant. Other signs of breast cancer you should be on the lookout for include:

- lumps near the underarm or armpit
- a nipple that suddenly inverts
- bloody discharge from the nipple
- puckering in the breast's skin
- other skin changes in the breast area, including red, swollen, and/or scaly patches

As we all know by now, outcomes for breast cancer patients are significantly better when the cancer is caught in the early stages. So keep up with your breast checks both at home and with your doctor after pregnancy as well.

DOWN THERE

>>> If you've never looked "down there" with purpose, now is the time to make nice with your nether region—*before* you get too big to bend over (and get real: it's going to happen). Try to scope out the scene so you'll know if something starts to look or feel weird during your pregnancy or after giving birth. You'll also be better equipped to ask for help in fixing the problem.

You've probably been misusing the word *vagina*. What we generally refer to as our vagina is more accurately our vulva, which comprises all the visible external organs down there, including your labia, clitoris, and pubic mound, as well as the openings to your urethra and your vagina. *Vagina* is just another name for the birth canal, the passageway that connects your external vulva to your womb (uterus).

Stabbing Crotch Pain

Does it sometimes feel as if lightning is striking your crotch, or like someone is stabbing you in your groin or pelvic area? While most pain in pregnancy is not normal, you shouldn't be alarmed by every single sudden twinge. A common cause of these shooting pains is your expanding uterus, which can cramp as it makes room for baby. Also, because your digestive system is out of whack, these pains may be a result of the excess gas or flatulence that's finding its way out.

Toward the end of your pregnancy, whether it's because of cervical dilation, baby's kicks, or nerve pain, it can sometimes feel as if your baby is kicking you in the crotch. So long as these episodes last for only a few seconds at a time, you'll probably be able to get through the pain with deep, controlled breaths.

That said, you should always mention any pain to your doctor, but especially if the pain is

- isolated to one side;
- more frequent than usual;
- extremely severe (such that it's hard for you to speak or breathe);
- and/or combined with fever, vaginal bleeding, or unusual discharge.

Those last symptoms can point to a more serious problem—or even the onset of labor. Call your doctor ASAP.

Swollen Vulva

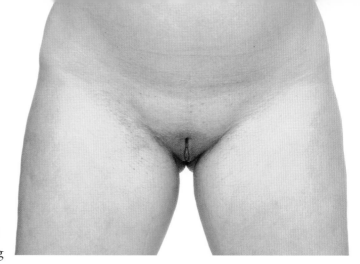

You're not imagining it if parts of your crotch, such as your labia, seem to be expanding. The swelling might be uneven, preferring one side, and it may come and go. It can even be painful. Whether the cause is edema (see page 2), pressure from your growing baby, or one of the myriad other possible issues, the day you discover any newfound developments down there can be truly terrifying. Read on to know what could happen and what you should do about it.

Varicose Veins Of the Vulva

First the good news: Your vulva hasn't magically sprouted new veins. Now for the bad news: Pregnancy has morphed your existing veins into gigantic vulvar varicosities, also known as

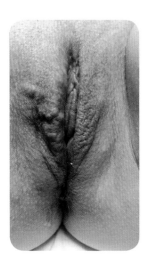

varicose veins of the vulva. Most women never realize they have varicose veins, but those who do find it difficult to forget about them because they are a source of pain and discomfort while sitting, standing, or walking (basically, most of the time!).

Vulvar varicosities are literally like having a hemorrhoid on your coochie, except Preparation H is no match for these meanies. The two conditions are somewhat related, though, because straining on the toilet due to constipation is a common cause of vulvar varicosities (and hemorrhoids; see page 61).

While vulvar varicosities may interfere with your general comfort, they probably won't affect your ability to have a normal vaginal delivery, and the veins usually shrink back down soon after birth.

HOW TO ⇨ Reduce Vulvar Swelling

Along with the suggestions on page 16 for everyday varicose veins, which can pop up elsewhere on your body, try these tips specifically to calm down your crotch:

- **Put it on ice.** Just like when your boobs are hurting (see page 38), placing a bag of frozen peas or corn down there can provide tremendous relief, and these bags conform to your body better than a regular (read: hard-as-a-rock) ice pack.
- **Get a vulvar girdle.** Spanx for your snatch are special support garments that really do exist (see the pictures below). They may look ridiculous, but they help to not only improve the comfort of existing vulvar varicosities but also lower your chances of developing new ones. These girdles go by other names like "V2" or "cradle," so you may have to do a little sleuthing to find them. But if you find something that looks like a modified jock strap and has decent reviews, snatch it up–it's what you're looking for.
- **Prop a pillow between your legs.** Do this whenever you are lying down on your side and before going to sleep to help relieve some of the positional pressure.

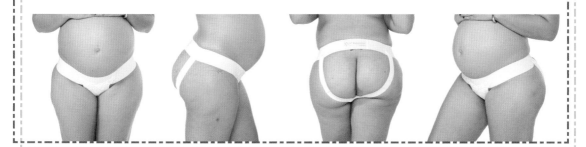

If your nether region seems a bit blue (in color, of course, not emotionally), you're not imagining things. Before the invention of pee sticks, doctors used to declare a woman pregnant based on a blue tint in the cervix, labia, and vagina, a condition known as Chadwick's sign. This is cause for celebration, not concern! However, if the lips on your face are turning blue, that is cause for concern; see page 109 for more info.

Pee Problems

Nearly all women will have some type of urinary issue during pregnancy, including urge incontinence, the medical term for those all-of-a-sudden times that you involuntarily pee (just a little) when laughing, coughing, sneezing, or exercising, among other regular activities. Being tethered to the toilet because of urge incontinence begins early in most pregnancies, and there's little you can do to control the frequency of those urges—now is certainly not the time to limit fluids. In fact, women who pee more often tend to have less of a problem with leaks than those who hold their urine and pee only a few times a day.

You'll want to do everything you can now to be sure that stress incontinence doesn't follow you for too long in the postpartum months. That means starting pelvic-floor exercises now (see page 53). Admittedly, I was a desperate dripper myself, and while everything eventually snapped back into place down there a few months after giving birth, I was in adult diapers for longer than I care to remember. I'd like to think that the pelvic-floor exercises are what saved the day in the long run, and hopefully, they will do the same for you.

On the bright side, most women see improvement shortly after giving birth, especially first-time mothers in their twenties and early thirties. However, weight gain, diet, and genetics play a part as well. Many women suffer silently in shame for years after giving birth, unaware that there is help available in the form of physical therapy and, in more severe cases, surgery. There's always hope!

Adult diapers are not just reserved for the old folks' home. They also happen to be one of the best-kept secrets among expecting and new moms. Once you get past the idea of wearing a diaper, you'll realize that modern versions are extremely discreet: they're also much better than wetting your panties, peeing on furniture, having an accident in public, or flooding the bed after a nighttime sneeze. Adult diapers will also come in handy after delivery, when your lochia—or bloody discharge from your lady parts—will be flowing. Pick up a bunch of packs and thank me later!

HOW TO ⇨ Perform Pelvic-floor Exercises

When done right, pelvic-floor muscle training can significantly reduce the effects of stress incontinence, both before and after delivery, by strengthening the reflexes of weakened tissues and muscles that can lead to urinary leakage.

Kegels are the most common exercises, and they are easy to do during pregnancy. Start on the toilet at first: When urinating, try to stop the flow for ten seconds before releasing, and repeat this action several times. Once you get the hang of it, you can do Kegels just about anywhere, and anytime (but without the peeing part!). Most experts recommend performing Kegels as often as possible throughout the day and, at a minimum, to complete at least three daily sets of ten to twenty repetitions for noticeable improvement.

You'll most likely need to work up to this amount over time, and it's better to start slow and make sure your technique is accurate—quality over quantity is essential to success. Squeezing the wrong muscles, such as those in your butt or legs rather than in your private parts, can hinder your progress. If you're having problems isolating the correct muscles to squeeze, don't be afraid to ask your doctor to help you—it's worth any embarrassment in the long run!

After all, a strong pelvic floor doesn't just improve incontinence. It can also increase your enjoyment of sex and lead to more powerful orgasms. (You're most welcome!)

She's laughing and not peeing on herself because she does Kegels!

53

Burning Pee (Infections)

Urinary tract infections (UTIs), or bladder infections, are a common occurrence during pregnancy because the bladder has the unfortunate problem of having to withstand the expanding uterus, which sits right on top of it. As the uterus grows, the weight can cause a blockage within the drainage system of the bladder. In this scenario, urine can get backed up and lead to an infection.

If you suspect you have an infection, you'll want to get tested and treated immediately by your doctor. If allowed to spread to the kidneys, which is also common in pregnancy, these infections will be much more serious. Kidney infections can result in hospitalization and can put you at risk for preterm labor and low birth weight. Signs that indicate you might have an infection include the following:

- pain or a burning sensation when you pee
- the feeling that you absolutely cannot wait to pee once you have the urge
- mucus or blood in the urine
- cloudy or foul-smelling urine
- pain or cramping sensations in the abdomen or back
- tenderness in the lower pelvic area
- pain when having sex
- fever, chills, or unexplained sweating
- vomiting or nausea

If you are prescribed antibiotics, be sure to complete the treatment, even if you start to feel better before the course is complete. Otherwise, the infection could worsen or even return.

You can try and blame your mother for a lot of other things, but when it comes to your hemorrhoids, vaginal varicose veins, and even your stress incontinence, you may be onto something. If you're subject to these frustrating symptoms during pregnancy, there are several contributing factors, one of which is a genetic predisposition. (Just remember all the good things you inherited from your mom, too!)

Smelly Crotch

You heard it here first (odds are): Sometimes pregnancy really stinks. More specifically, your private parts can smell pretty gross at times, especially for the 65 percent of women who report a change in vaginal odor during pregnancy. I, sadly, was a card-carrying member of this pregnancy crotch rot, so trust me when I say you don't have to dig yourself a hole of shame to squat in for the remainder of your pregnancy—your super-sensitive nose is picking up way more scent than anyone else.

That doesn't mean that the change in the odor of your privates is all in your head. Hopefully, it's not an infection (see page 56). Typical reasons you're feeling (and smelling) not so fresh include a pregnancy-induced elevated vaginal pH, which not only changes your odor but also causes urinary incontinence (as discussed on page 52) as well as an increase in vaginal mucus, sweat, and other scent-sational secretions. Prenatal vitamins can also contribute to a stronger smell down there.

> One reason your body odor changes is that you're perspiring for two: You smell a little bit like the baby you're carrying. That's another reason why your urine smells funny, too—it's blended with that of the baby.

News flash: If you're suffering from an incredibly strong smell, your underwear, not your genitals, may be to blame. Pee, sweat, and other secretions collect in the crotch of your panties, and odors become trapped in the fibers, ripening into that singular gas-station-bathroom-floor smell. Changing your underwear (preferably cotton) as often as possible is an excellent idea. However, for those of us who haven't the room (or wherewithal) to keep five or six pairs of panties in our purses, protecting your underwear with a maxi-pad or panty liner that you change every couple of hours should significantly diminish the smell.

> Some women insist that eliminating certain foods also minimizes body funk. Common fiends for genital odor include garlic, sugar, caffeine, spicy foods, onions, and red meat. Talk with your doctor, however, before drastically changing your diet during pregnancy.

For true genital odors, use baby wipes to freshen up throughout the day—any packages left over will come in handy when baby is born.

Smelly Infections & STDs

Besides the annoying-yet-normal reasons for a smelly crotch described on page 55, you'll want to be on the lookout (or smell-out) for any abnormal causes, which require a doctor's appointment ASAP:

- **Infections.** If you're suffering from a smelly discharge plus itching, your problem might be bacterial vaginosis (BV) or a vaginal yeast infection (also known as vaginal thrush). Yeast infections crop up often in pregnancy, especially after taking an antibiotic. If you're simply dealing with an awful odor, a UTI or bladder infection may be the culprit (see page 54). If left untreated, an infection can lead to issues with preterm labor and even miscarriage.

- **Sexually transmitted diseases (STDs).** Herpes, trichomoniasis, chlamydia, gonorrhea, and other sexually transmitted diseases could also be the cause of your vaginal odor. Pregnancy often brings dormant diseases to the forefront, even if you've never had an outbreak before. And let's be frank and acknowledge the cold, hard facts: The looming reality of becoming a parent (and all that entails) can trigger a bout of infidelity by

> *A pregnant woman and her best friend are driving when they see a skunk with a wounded leg who is unable to get itself out of the road. They decide to take the skunk to the vet, so they bring it into the car and see that the skunk is shivering. The pregnant woman says, "The skunk is cold! What should we do?" The best friend replies, "Put it between your legs to keep it warm." The pregnant woman hesitates, saying "What about the smell?" Her best friend replies, "Hold its nose."*

even the most unlikely of partners, opening the door for STDs. (Just saying! See the *Sex & Love* section that starts on page 151 for more.)

If you have even the slightest concern that you might have an infection or an STD, do not avoid talking to your doctor out of fear of feeling ashamed. For starters, your doctor has for sure seen (and smelled) worse. Secondly, it's difficult, if not impossible, for you alone to sniff out whether your odor is unhealthy, so your doctor needs to run a few quick tests to rule out anything serious.

Douching: Just Say No

Pregnant or not, and no matter how frustrated you are by your distinctive funk, do not douche. Period. If you have an infection, douching will only serve to spread it. If you don't have an infection, douching will only worsen your pH-balance problem—and the odors that go along with that. Studies have also shown a correlation between douching during pregnancy and preterm births. You should stay away from so-called hygienic wipes, too, unless your doctor recommends them. These can be irritating to the skin and can actually lead to vaginal infection.

Leaky Vagina

Besides urine and normal discharge, pregnancy brings about leukorrhea, the medical term for the milky, mild-smelling, thin vaginal discharge that you may have noticed by now. Your very own "snail trail" is another of the earliest signs of pregnancy, and it becomes stronger and more noticeable as you get further along. This is good, because leukorrhea protects the vaginal canal against infection. However, watch out for a significant increase in discharge, which can be a sign of STDs (page 56), UTIs (page 54), or vaginal yeast infections (page 56). Wearing a light pad or panty liner can help manage the odor and discomfort from leakage. As always, be sure to discuss any change in your vaginal discharge with your doctor.

Nearly one-third of women will suffer from bacterial vaginosis at some point during pregnancy (myself included). While this condition isn't a sexually transmitted infection per se, it is a bacterial imbalance associated with vaginal intercourse. Your doctor can clear the infection (and, consequently, the air around your underwear).

Spotting In Early Pregnancy

About 25 percent of all mamas-to-be have some bleeding or spotting during the first trimester of pregnancy. Most of the time, this is completely harmless; in some cases, however, it can signal a problem with the pregnancy, and it is difficult to know the difference. Some causes of normal spotting in the first trimester include:

- sexual activity
- implantation spotting (when the embryo burrows into your uterus)
- cervical changes
- changes in pregnancy hormones

Always alert your doctor at the first sign of bleeding or spotting, and insist upon being seen if it happens more than once, as you will want to rule out any serious causes, including infections (sexual and nonsexual), ectopic pregnancy, molar pregnancy, or a miscarriage.

As your due date approaches, that kicking sensation in your belly is not, as you might think, the baby's way of letting you know he is ready for his debut. Most babies are already turned with their heads facing down by now. So even if a baby could kick his way out, his feet are in the wrong position to do so. What's really causing that knocking at your lady door is the pressure from the baby's head (or, in some cases, his feet or tushy) pushing its way down toward the birth canal, which in turn causes your cervix to dilate in preparation for labor and delivery.

Spotting In Later Pregnancy

In later pregnancy, you can have normal spotting or bleeding because of the following:

- early labor
- sexual activity
- cervical dilation
- a pelvic exam by your doctor

Serious causes of bleeding in late pregnancy include:

- placenta previa (where the placenta is overlying the cervix)
- premature labor
- placental separation (or abruption)
- rupture of the uterus

Again, you alone can't tell the difference between what's normal and what's not. Tell your doctor if you have spotting or bleeding at any point during your pregnancy so she can identify a problem—or hopefully just give you peace of mind.

Passing Gas

Pregnancy not only causes your body to create more gas, but also relaxes your anal muscles, making it harder to hold all that extra gas in and turning you into a farty, burping, and bloated mama-to-be.

Be prepared for your body to pass gas when you least expect it, whether it's in the middle of a board meeting or while enjoying your baby shower. Instead of being embarrassed, just shrug it off and blame the gas on being pregnant (which is true, so there!).

Aside from chewing your food thoroughly, eating smaller meals, and avoiding drinking with straws, there's really nothing you can do to prevent a gassy buildup until you give birth. Sure, you could also try limiting foods known to lead to belly bloat, but why bother? Isn't it much more important to have a healthy, well-balanced diet that nourishes both you and your baby?

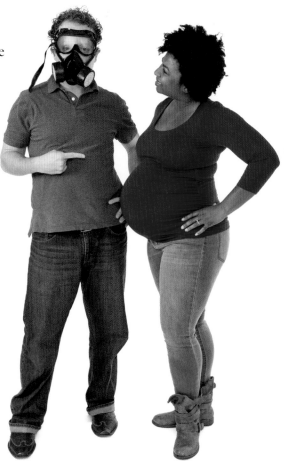

Constipation

Pregnant poop is no fun for the many women who suffer from constipation during this time. For starters, food is digested more slowly in pregnancy, and then there's your growing uterus that often presses on the rectum—both factors leading to constipation. Iron supplements also tend not to help matters.

Fortunately, there are things you can do to keep your bowel movements regular and pain free. Drinking more water and eating more fibrous foods (which you should be doing anyway and always) usually help the problem tremendously. Use caution when considering laxatives, even "natural" ones such as senna, as some types can cause uterine contractions and possibly encourage labor (castor oil is infamous for this). Ask your doctor about possible safe options, some of which may be available only by prescription.

Hemorrhoids

Constipation can lead to hemorrhoids, which are a type of varicose vein located in the anus. Hemorrhoids can be uncomfortable and itchy or downright painful. About half of all pregnant women will develop hemorrhoids. To keep them at bay, do any (or all) of the following:

- **Kegel exercises.** These will strengthen the pelvic muscles. See page 53.
- **Sleep on your side.** It's better for hemorrhoids than sleeping on your back.
- **Avoid straining when pooping.** Take your time, don't rush, and let gravity help you.
- **Clean thoroughly after pooping.** Keep your anal area as hygienic as possible to avoid irritation. Baby wipes are your trusted friends.
- **Ice the itchy spots.** Tuck ice packs (or frozen veggies; see page 39), or a panty pad soaked in witch hazel, between your buttocks to alleviate the itches that you shouldn't scratch.
- **Sit on a doughnut-shaped pillow.** Resting your tushy on one of these special cushions will help reduce the pressure there.
- **Drink lots of water.** As mentioned before, dehydration is a common culprit in hemorrhoid-causing constipation.

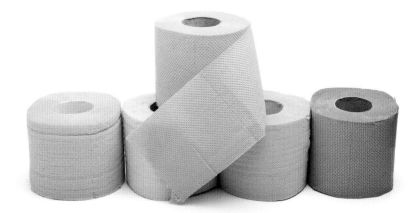

 What do you call a pregnant woman who won't fart in front of her partner? A private tooter!

Diarrhea

You can suffer from diarrhea during pregnancy due to any number of reasons, including:

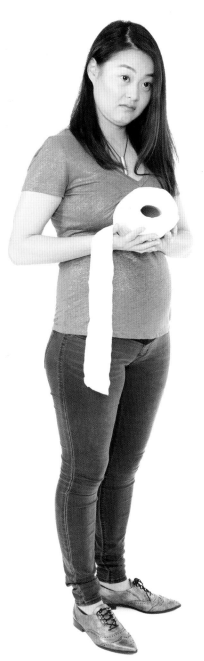

- changes in your diet
- food sensitivities (these often crop up during pregnancy)
- prenatal vitamins
- hormonal changes

As you get closer to your delivery date, you might experience more frequent episodes of diarrhea, as these are often considered to be the body's way of clearing the path for the baby during labor. But don't be in a rush to pack your hospital bags: Having beyond-normal diarrhea doesn't always mean you're ready to go into labor, at least not yet!

See your doctor if you have diarrhea that doesn't go away after two or three days. Never take over-the-counter medicine without your doctor's recommendation. Antidiarrheal medication can worsen some of the conditions that are causing diarrhea in the first place.

The "down there" of your fetus isn't distinguishable for the first couple of months, which is why it takes so long to determine the baby's gender. Starting in the third month, the genital tubercle forms into a penis or a clitoris—which will be visible on the ultrasound, so cover your eyes if you don't want to spoil the surprise!

ACHES
& PAINS

> You conquered your morning sickness (at last!). You tamed your emotional roller coaster (bravo!). Now for your next hurdle: your aching body! Pregnancy can be a pain in the butt—literally and figuratively. Read on to figure out what's normal and what's not.

Cramping

Watch out for any cramping after the first few weeks of pregnancy. Before then, it's common to experience cramping when the fertilized egg attaches itself to the uterine wall. And mild cramping is par for the course as your uterus expands and all the other internal organs smoosh together. But if the cramping is steady or intense, you should discuss it immediately with your doctor.

Contractions

Pregnancy is a big deal for your body. It's a time when your abdominal, uterine, and vaginal muscles can really shine. Besides, when else do they all get to work together as a team? As with any respectable team, these muscles are going to engage in a few friendly practice games (i.e., contractions) before the main event.

Most expectant mothers experience three types of contractions during their pregnancy, including (in order of both appearance and pain): "We're here! We kind of know what we're doing!" contractions (a.k.a. Braxton Hicks); followed by "Put us in, coach! We're warmed up and ready!" contractions (a.k.a. false contractions); and lastly, "We're in this to win!" contractions (a.k.a. real contractions, as in Get Ready).

Braxton Hicks contractions, named after the doctor who discovered them after studying a lot of pregnant women who were worried about preterm labor, can kick in any time during your pregnancy, but many women begin having them during the second trimester and into the third. These contractions are irregular and unpredictable, and there's not much you can do about them except to stay calm and try to breathe through the discomfort. They're more uncomfortable than painful, and tend to naturally dial themselves down instead of ratcheting up. They're another reason to drink up, too—dehydration is thought to be a contributing cause.

False contractions can begin several weeks, days, or hours before the real deal, and serve to nudge the cervix into the "ready zone," though they don't necessarily lead to dilation. They're considered *false* because they are characterized as being intermittent and will stop when you shift positions.

Real contractions hurt. You'll know when you're having them. Their function is to help dilate the cervix. After all, you're about to push a melon through a lemon-size portal, and these contractions are your body's way of preparing you to do just that. Real contractions are rhythmic and powerful. Sometimes they'll take your breath away, so repeat after me: inhale, exhale, inhale, exhale. Besides a punch-in-the-gut sensation, each contraction is typically accompanied by pain in your lower back, thighs, and abs. Brace yourself.

Oh, and at some point (either before or during real contractions), your water will break. Anecdotally, these get-ready contractions are stronger if the water breaks before they start. I can attest to this painful truth. Hang in there—you'll make it to the finish line yet!

Belly & Round Ligament Pain

The round ligaments that support the uterus stretch during pregnancy to provide support for your growing baby. Sometimes they spasm, which can cause sharp, jablike pains in the lower belly or groin. Round ligament pains are only felt for a few seconds at a time, and offer no real cause for concern. Sneezing, laughing, coughing, and other everyday actions can trigger them, so consider yourself forewarned.

Upper Right Tummy Pain? Not Normal!

An intense pain on the right side of your belly should never be ignored. Not only is it a sign of preeclampsia (see page 4 for more), but also it is not uncommon to need surgery in pregnancy for appendicitis or acute cholecystitis. Acute cholecystitis in pregnant women is most often caused by an impacted gallstone in the cystic duct. While pregnant women tend to have gallstones more than other people, this fact alone is not related to an increased risk for developing cholecystitis.

Acute cholecystitis and related gallbladder issues cause severe pain in the upper right quadrant and may be accompanied by jaundice, fever, nausea, vomiting, and pain or diarrhea after eating fatty foods. Appendicitis produces intense pain in the lower right quadrant as well as nausea and vomiting paired with a fever.

There is nothing you can do to prevent these medical issues from cropping up (either before, during, or after pregnancy), but there is absolutely something you can do if you are experiencing abdominal pain: Call your doctor at once! Delaying treatment could just worsen the problem and lead to further complications. Diagnosis is quick and easy, and if warranted, you can explore a course of treatment.

Diastasis Recti

If you feel a pulling, burning pain where your abs once were (or where you always wished they were), chances are you're dealing with diastasis recti. Don't be put off by the medical jargon. *Diastasis* is Latin for separation, and *recti* means abdominals. Basically, your abs split apart, straight down the middle, into two parts on either side of connective tissue that goes by the name of linea alba. Although it sounds scary, diastasis recti is a perfectly normal occurrence—most mamas will experience this stomach separation.

Many women are able to bounce back from diastasis recti, while lots of others have this issue to blame for their perpetual "mummy tummy" that tends to stick around—especially after a second or third (or fourth . . .) pregnancy—despite any amount of diet or exercise.

Aesthetics aside, having a split stomach is problematic because you need your abs for more than strutting a bikini body. A weakened core affects your day-to-day capacity by limiting your stamina and strength. Sufferers of diastasis recti are also prone to postpartum umbilical hernias.

You can certainly try using some strategically placed kinetic tape (as shown below) or a pregnancy belly support to lower your odds (and to relieve pressure from your growing tummy), but diastasis recti can happen to anyone—though hopefully not to you!

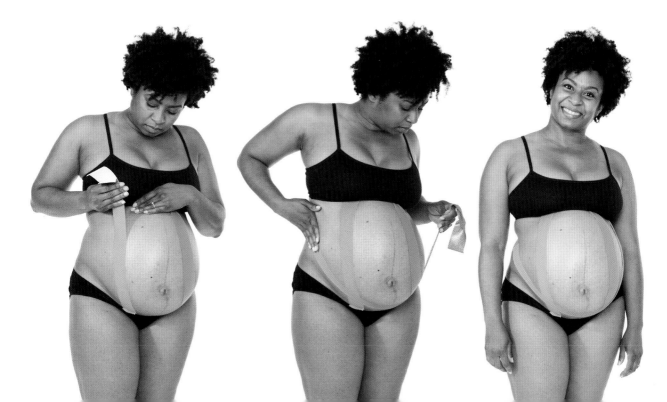

Take Pelvic Girdle Pain Seriously!

Sciatica can sometimes be felt in your pelvis, but pain in this area more often stems from pelvic girdle pain, or PGP for short. PGP is common (it's what's behind the telltale "pregnancy waddle") but all too often underestimated. It can involve a whole other level of back pain, plus complications that should be taken seriously.

The pelvic area includes your hip bones, tailbone, and sacrum along with a handful of joints, including the symphysis pubis—a potentially big part of your pain and suffering (people used to refer to PGP as symphysis pubis dysfunction, or SPD). As the ligaments and muscles in the region loosen, the joints of the pelvis can become unstable and often misaligned as your baby grows and needs more space.

> Pelvic pain often strikes in the postpartum months, too, even if you didn't have it during pregnancy. Be aware of the signs and symptoms and discuss them with your doctor if you feel this might be happening to you.

This misalignment makes itself known in several ways. Typical symptoms in the early stages include hearing and feeling popping or clicking sensations in the pelvic area, and you'll likely experience discomfort when engaging the hip and pelvic muscles; in other words, you'll notice PGP when sitting, standing, and walking (so pretty much all the time), and even during sex, if you're still having it.

Hopefully the sound (and sensation) of snap, crackle, pop (!) is all the trouble your pelvis gives you during pregnancy, but some sufferers find that PGP leaves them completely incapacitated. Think of a marionette whose strings suddenly go lax and all the wooden parts start bumping into each other. This loosening of the muscles and ligaments that's at the root of PGP is designed to help with delivery, but until that day finally happens, PGP can be a tremendous pain in the butt.

Unlike other types of back pain that can be relieved or improved with gentle exercises, these and other movements can aggravate the already severe PGP symptoms. For this reason, acute cases of PGP can be nightmarish for active pregnant women, who are often expected to just "push through" the pain like everyone else—and who often end up feeling anxious or depressed on top of having to live in tremendous discomfort. PGP can create a financial burden, too, especially if the mom is put on bed rest and is unable to work.

Whatever you do, don't give in to societal pressure! Ignoring the pain is not good for your current or long-term health, and you could end up with disc problems and chronic pain that last long after birth.

One source of relief you may want to try is called a vulvar girdle (see page 51 for more on this device, shown opposite). It is rather ridiculous looking, but often effective. You can purchase a vulvar girdle online or at many prenatal physical therapist offices.

Here are a few additional ways to help alleviate the pain on your own:

- when lying down, turn on your side as much as possible, using pillows for support
- when sitting, choose chairs that provide ample back support
- when standing or walking, watch your posture and keep your knees close together to limit pelvic stress

Finally, you may not be able to control the reactions of your friends and coworkers, but if your doctor doesn't take your pain levels seriously, find one who does. And if no one else believes you, know that I do!

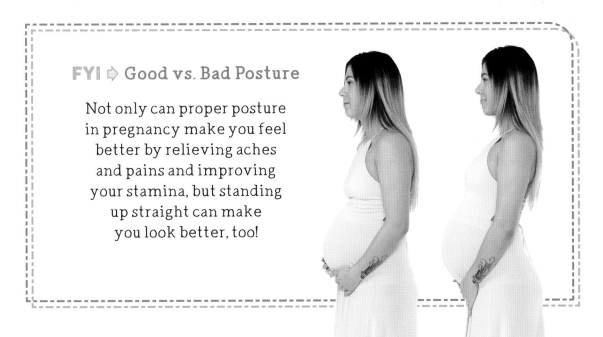

FYI ➩ Good vs. Bad Posture

Not only can proper posture in pregnancy make you feel better by relieving aches and pains and improving your stamina, but standing up straight can make you look better, too!

BACKACHES

Whether it's because of stress, hormones, or strain from your ever-growing baby bump (or all of the above), most mamas-to-be report back pain at some point during their pregnancy.

Lower Back Pain

Lower back pain, also known as lumbar pain, can be present much earlier in pregnancy than pain in your upper back. Indeed, it is often one of the first signs that you're a mama-to-be! Your lower back might hurt all the time or only when you do certain activities, like climbing stairs or vigorous exercising. Staying in one position for long periods of time, whether sitting or standing, can make the pain worse. Acupuncture of the ear has been proven effective at helping pregnant women manage lower back pain; wearing a pregnancy-specific back brace and doing gentle exercise also helps.

Upper Back Pain

Upper back pain usually doesn't start until later in pregnancy, when your (and your baby's) weight gain starts to really take its toll. If your breasts have grown especially big, they might be to blame; besides pulling your shoulders down, their weight puts more stress and strain on your shoulders and neck. Your best bet is to stow away your sexy lingerie and get fitted for a super-supportive "boulder holder" (like those giant bras in vintage cartoons).

If the pain in your upper back is limited to just one side and is accompanied by fever or painful urination, this may be a sign that you have a kidney infection (see page 54)—and your cue to alert your doctor ASAP.

Sciatica

If along with your lower back pain you feel pain in your buttocks, legs, or feet (whether both sides or just one side), that special form of torture is called sciatica. The longest, largest nerve in your body is the sciatic nerve, and it's located behind the uterus and travels down your legs. When the baby—along with your blossoming placenta and uterus—puts pressure on this nerve, it can cause bouts of severe pain that radiate up and down your bottom half. Resting on your side as well as performing Kegel exercises (page 53) and yoga (see page 77) can help you manage the pain, along with doctor-approved pain medication.

If you ever have back pain—or to avoid ever having it in the first place—wearing comfy sneakers should be a shoo-in (or make that shoe-in!). High heels can further throw your body's balance off and worsen any back pain, while many flats and flip-flops just don't stack up when it comes to providing support.

HEADACHES

If it's any consolation, studies show that four out of five pregnant women have headaches, so you're certainly in good company if you're one of these sufferers. In fact, headaches are frequently one of the first pregnancy symptoms to show up, and being with child gives them a unique spin, especially because you can't just pop pain medicine like you used to—many seemingly harmless meds, even OTC options, can be problematic for baby. In particular, aspirin, ibuprofen, and other nonsteroidal anti-inflammatory drugs are not recommended in pregnancy.

If headaches are a constant refrain throughout your pregnancy, they're most likely just annoying rather than harmful. However, if you suddenly start having headaches in your third trimester, or if your third-trimester headaches are unlike the ones you've been having all along, call your doctor ASAP—these new or different headaches could be a sign of preeclampsia, a serious complication discussed on page 4.

Tension Headaches

Tension headaches are the most common type to crop up during pregnancy, and they generally feel like a dull ache that is spread evenly over your head. The surge of estrogen in pregnancy can be a trigger, as can the increase in blood volume. But stress, caffeine withdrawal, and/or dehydration—all typical aspects of baby-growing—can also be culprits.

Migraines

Around 20 percent of pregnant women suffer from migraine headaches, which feel entirely different—and can be much more debilitating—than other types. The pain is usually stronger by far, sticks to one side of your head, and gets worse with movement and exposure to light.

Tell your doctor if you begin having migraines on a regular basis. Pregnant women who suffer from migraines have a much higher risk of developing preeclampsia.

If you're dealing with migraines in your first trimester, take comfort in knowing that between 50 and 70 percent of women see an improvement in later trimesters. Fingers crossed! Meanwhile, you can try and pinpoint the possible triggers, including your sleep cycle as well as certain odors or foods. MSG, artificial sweeteners, and nitrates are common culprits you might want to avoid consuming.

Keeping a detailed sleep, activity, and dietary journal for a few days can also be a big help. You may want to talk to your doctor about magnesium supplements or infusions, too, as these can be effective at preventing or treating migraines.

Sinus Headaches

Sinus headaches might also be bringing you down, and you have progesterone—an important pregnancy hormone that can cause swelling in the sinus linings and an increase in mucus production—to thank for that. This type of headache can also be caused by rhinitis (if you're sneezy and itchy), sinusitis (if your eyes, upper cheeks, and forehead are painful), or your basic head cold (if you just feel miserable).

If you were addicted to coffee or soda before pregnancy and have been cutting your caffeine intake down, your headaches might be caused by caffeine withdrawal.

Restless Leg Syndrome

If your legs seem to have minds of their own when you lie down these days, and you have the frustrating sensation of needing to keep moving them because they're burning or itching or twanging, then you may have a sleep disorder called restless leg syndrome (or RLS).

RLS in pregnancy is sometimes caused by an iron or folate deficiency, so if you haven't been taking your prenatal vitamins, you're probably kicking yourself right now—at least while in bed. If you are taking your vitamins, talk to your doctor about increasing the dosage. You can also get more of these essential nutrients through a carefully planned diet.

Leg Cramping

Painful, unpredictable muscle tightening in your legs can literally cramp your style. Like restless leg syndrome, leg cramps, also known as "charley horses," often happen at night and can ruin any chance of getting a good night's sleep. If you start to feel a cramp coming on, immediately straighten your leg and start flexing your foot, heel to toe, to try and stretch the muscle.

Even better, you can prevent the cramps from happening in the first place by stretching out your legs before you hit the hay. Standing about a foot away from a wall, and keeping the soles of your feet flat on the floor, lean forward with your arms outstretched and your palms placed against the wall. Hold for five to ten seconds, give yourself a break, and repeat ten times.

If your leg pain is one-sided and/or accompanied by swelling, talk to your doctor about the possibility of deep vein thrombosis (DVT), which is a blood clotting issue not uncommon in pregnancy.

Weak Ankles

No one is stronger than a mother, yet there's nothing weaker than a mother-to-be's ankles. To prepare for baby's grand exit, your body produces relaxin, the hormone that wins the Most Aptly Named contest and that, well, relaxes the ligaments in your body. Unfortunately, relaxin doesn't have very specific aim and, as a result, your ankles become weaklings. Combine that with your added weight and shifting center of gravity and you've got yourself a perfect storm for suffering a twisted ankle (or two or four or eight). I should know: I twisted my ankles so many times while pregnant that I had to stop taking the subway for fear I might fall onto the train tracks!

The only thing you can really do to avoid a similar fate is to wear supportive shoes, preferably ones that cushion the ankle (anyone for high-tops?) and/or to wear ankle supports. You should also walk consciously, keeping a careful eye out for uneven spots in the sidewalk or other potential hazards that may be lurking. Avoid hurrying whenever possible. And remember: Your weak ankles won't affect your baby in the slightest, but doing a belly flop on the ground just might. Should this fate befall (sorry!) you, proceed directly to your doctor's office or the nearest hospital to have everything checked out.

Physical Therapy For Pain

If your back pain is interfering with your ability to function normally at work and at home, your doctor can prescribe physical therapy. In these sessions, a trained professional will show you some targeted stretches to help pinpoint and alleviate your problems—and, when appropriate, give you a soothing massage to relax the muscles. Most insurance policies also cover acupuncture treatments (sometimes without requiring a referral), so the solution to your back pain may just be a co-pay away!

HOW TO ⇨ Soothe Aches and Pains Safely

As a mom-to-be, you can no longer pop any pill that's worked for your aches and pains in the past. Specifically, you should never take ibuprofen, naproxen, aspirin, or any other OTC remedy not approved by your doctor. Keep in mind: While your headaches won't affect the baby, some medications just might. Ask your doctor about taking acetaminophen (such as Tylenol), which is usually OK.

In lieu of painkillers, mix peppermint or another minty essential oil together with coconut or olive oil and ask your partner to massage this potion onto your temples, scalp, neck, shoulder, back, leg, or any other painful areas. Not only will this hands-on treatment feel wonderfully relaxing, but the essential oils have a cooling effect that can help soothe aches.

If your pain becomes unbearable, your doctor may be able to provide a pregnancy-safe prescription.

Massage Pressure Points That Are Off-limits

It's safest to see only certified prenatal massage therapists when pregnant, since there are certain pressure points that can induce contractions and preterm labor. But sometimes it's just too hard to pass up a quick rubdown with your mani-pedi or when shopping at the mall. Just make sure that whoever's giving you the massage knows you're expecting—and be prepared to call it quits when and if he rubs you in these spots, which should always be avoided during pregnancy:

- the area around your wrists
- the area between your index finger and thumb
- the area around your ankles
- the arch of your foot

Of course, if you're getting a massage in your forty-second week, by all means rub away at these pressure points—and good luck getting that baby out ASAP!

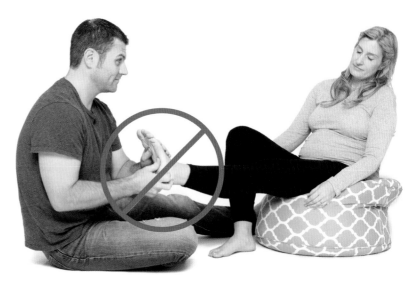

Massage is good for not just you but also baby! In multiple studies, women who received twice weekly massages during pregnancy (either from a partner or a professional) had babies that were not only calmer in utero but also way less likely to be born prematurely!

HOW TO ⇨ Do Prenatal Yoga

If you've been hitting the mat for years, feel free to continue with yoga once you're pregnant. If you've never tried it before, there's no time like the present. Several yoga poses specifically target your pelvic and back muscles. Why bother with stretching your pelvis? Many studies show that pelvic stretches help to fix or improve everything from pregnancy-related incontinence to lower back pain.

Aside from yoga's many physical benefits, the breath work will help keep you calm and centered—two qualities often in short supply during pregnancy and labor. You can conveniently practice these pregnancy-approved poses in your own home (thanks, Internet!) or be social and find a prenatal yoga class. You'll appreciate the community of support as well as the pregnancy-adapted poses. If you take a regular yoga class, unless it's obvious, be sure and tell the instructor that you're pregnant so she can ensure you're doing the poses safely.

And despite your proficiency, not all yoga poses are safe during pregnancy, including these to avoid: inverted poses, full wheel pose, deep forward bends, and anything you don't feel comfortable doing. Also, skip hot yoga until after birth. Namaste!

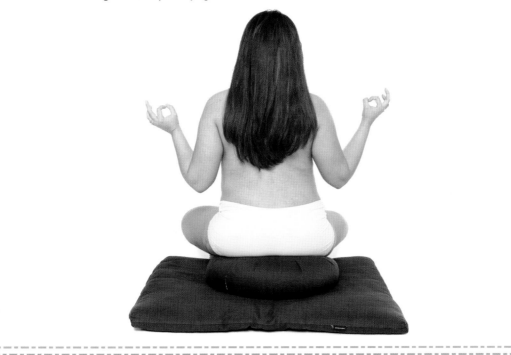

Facial Numbness & Paralysis

A pregnant woman's body has a life of its own (beyond the baby growing inside), yet you may be surprised to discover that even simple facial expressions and sensations can become difficult to control. Don't fall into a panic and mistake any sudden facial numbness or paralysis for a stroke; there are a couple of less frightening, and more likely, explanations that stem from your pregnancy.

Migraines, for example, can have the terrifying side effect of temporary numbness in your face, as can nerve damage, which is also a major cause of pregnancy-related Bell's palsy. This latter condition is described as a numbing sensation, twitching, or paralysis in one or both sides of the face, including the eyelids and mouth, which may also droop.

Talk to your doctor ASAP if you have any cause for concern. If left untreated, Bell's palsy can have unfortunate and permanent side effects, including blindness if it affects your eyelids. With proper treatment, however, these possibilities are much slimmer. Although most women find that the symptoms go away after delivery, any damage done during pregnancy could pose problems long afterward. That's why it is important to tell your doctor now.

Ask your doctor to check your vitamin levels to see if there's a nutritional deficiency that could be to blame for your symptoms. Devising a long-term treatment plan now rather than later can also help ease your mind, improve the prognosis, and reduce the risk of permanent damage, especially if you have Bell's palsy. If you don't feel that your doctor is taking you seriously, you may want to ask for a referral to a physical therapist, or find a different doctor who better respects your concerns.

Always tell your doctor if you experience numbness or paralysis of any kind, whether it's in your legs, arms, or other body parts—but especially in your face. Facial numbness in pregnancy can occasionally be a symptom of stroke, preeclampsia, or even herpes. And even if your paralysis is a temporary pregnancy problem, it can follow you into the postpartum phase and even worsen over time.

NOSE

Nose Growth

Whether your swollen sniffer is subtle or super-obvious, there are a few reasons why this development is happening to you at this particular time, including:

- **Enlarged mucous membranes.** Pregnancy expands these types of membranes throughout your body, including those in your nose.
- **Weight gain.** Some noses have more fatty tissue than others, especially around the tip, and this tissue can expand just like a midriff "muffin top" when you gain weight—which you're doing a lot of while baking a baby.
- **Extra blood and plasma.** Some of those added pounds of fluid that come with pregnancy might be hanging around your nose, causing it to be more notable.

Remember that this, like many bodily changes, won't be nearly as noticeable to others as it is to you. Should you start having trouble breathing or experiencing other nose-related problems, call your doctor—these may or may not be related to your nose growth.

Odds are, your nasal swelling is merely cosmetic and only temporary. As your body adjusts to postpartum life, your snout will likely shrink back to its previous size. If it doesn't, some doctors attribute that to lingering pregnancy weight, so think about whether your schnozzle is the only part of your body that's still on the plus side.

Nosebleeds

Your vagina won't be needing a tampon for the next few months, but your snout just might! If you're already prone to nosebleeds, you can expect to have even more while you're expecting. If you've never experienced them, get ready—your nose's many tiny blood vessels often get cranky with pregnancy's increased blood volume and decide to mimic a volcano erupting all over your shirt!

If (when) you experience a nosebleed, try to sit down immediately. First, gently blow your nose, and then, keeping your head above your heart, lean slightly forward (so blood pours out of your nose and not down your throat) while gently pinching your nostrils together with your thumb and forefinger and remain in this position for fifteen minutes. If you are still bleeding by now, go to your nearest emergency room for an evaluation. Either way, once the bleeding stops, call your doctor for a follow-up appointment.

You can also help prevent nosebleeds from happening by using only gentle force when blowing your nose—the more you huff and puff, the more your nostrils might bleed away. Running humidifiers in your house, especially in your bedroom while you sleep, also helps by keeping your mucous membranes from becoming too dry.

Worried about your nose job surviving your pregnancy? Rhinoplasty is mainly performed on bone and cartilage. In contrast, pregnancy swelling happens in the surrounding tissues—so your beautified beak should not be permanently affected.

TRUE STORY:
I HATED MY HUSBAND'S SMELL!

BY CHAUNIE BRUSIE, RN, BSN

Here's the scene: I'm standing at the kitchen stove sautéing carrots and onions while trying not to gag right into the pan. But it isn't my morning sickness (OK, fine, fine, "24/7 sickness") that turns my stomach and makes me cringe. The real problem? My husband. More specifically, my husband's smell.

The sad and unfortunate truth is that when I'm pregnant, my husband suddenly smells a bit peculiar to me. And by *peculiar*, I mean I kind of sort of can't stand the smell of him. Before you start thinking I'm a horrible person, allow me to assure you that I love my husband. I think he's a wonderful partner and an even better father. He's the kind of guy I hoped to find when I was a young girl dreaming about my future, the kind who cooks us pancakes on the weekends, makes my kids laugh that deep belly laugh when he throws them into the air (and that I can never get them to do), and folds T-shirts into tiny little squares as if he spent years in retail. The point is my husband is the Real Deal. That doesn't change the fact that I can't stand to be near him when I'm pregnant.

I'm sure there's probably some kind of biological, hormonal, or physiological reason for the fact that during the fifteen months (OK, fine, fine,

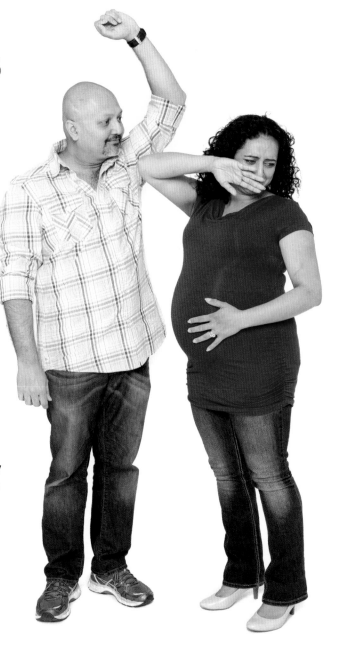

ten months) that I'm pregnant, catching a whiff of my husband's musky man-scent turns my stomach. But honestly, I'm too busy trying to silently puke in the corner before he notices to investigate the reasons behind my olfactory struggles.

Because really, how do you tell your beloved husband, protector, and soul mate, and the father of your child, that for some strange reason, growing his baby also means a growing disgust for him? I just go with it and accept either that I'm the world's worst wife or that pregnancy is just a weird, weird time that does weird, weird things to some of us. Some women get cravings, some women deal with a change in their sense of smell, and some others apparently experience odor aversions that strangely affect only how their husbands smell to them.

The point is, I've been pregnant four times now and each time I have experienced a lot of different symptoms, but this one has regrettably been a constant source of dismay (much like my stretch marks and pregnancy pouch). No matter what I do or how hard I try to will it away, I still can't shake the fact that my husband just smells different to me when I'm preggers.

The good news is, if you too suffer from I-hate-my-husband's-smell-when-I'm-pregnantitis, the condition is only temporary. My affliction literally has gone away minutes after I've given birth, which may or may not be related to the fact that my husband brings something delicious for me to eat when I've just burned a million and a half calories having a baby–and is suddenly more attractive than ever.

YOU'RE PREGNANT! A.K.A.

Gravid * In Pig * Harboring a Fugitive * Stung By a Serpent * Baking a Baby * In Happy Circumstances * Baby Farming * Spawning * With Child * Swole Up * Infanticipating * Knocked Up * In a Family Way * Smuggling a Basketball * Incubating * Fermenting * Growing a Watermelon * In Cyesis * In a Fix * Enlarged * Up the Duff * Fishing Out a Trout In the Well * Preggers * Preggo * Sprouting a Bean * Eating For Two * Wearing the Bustle Wrong * Great Bellied * Shucking a Pea In Your Pod * Heavy

Funky Smells

If many aspects of your pregnancy are starting to stink, take a deep breath (through your mouth, not your nose!). You're just among the two-thirds of preggos who experience hyperosmia, an increased ability to perceive odors. Scientists aren't positive what's behind this sense sensitivity, but it can show itself in what I call the Four *A*'s:

- **Awareness.** Many pregnant women notice an increase in the number—and power—of the smells they detect (from their own genitals to freshly cut grass).
- **Aversion.** Smells that previously were easy to ignore, or just slightly irritating, sometimes become gag-inducing (like cigarette smoke or cat poop).
- **Attraction.** Some women admit to actually craving and seeking out certain smells while pregnant, from taking a whiff of mud to sniffing fabric softener. (See page 133 for how this plays out with food cravings.)
- **Assumed.** Over 10 percent of pregnant women find themselves smelling odors that aren't even there, a phenomenon called "phantom smells."

Aside from being annoying, your heightened sense of smell can affect your appetite, nausea levels, mobility (since you may find yourself feeling sick when confronted with so many persistent odors), and personal self-esteem—especially if you, like pregnant me, think you're suffering from a constant case of crotch rot (as described on page 55).

> **Baby's eyesight might be blurry for the first few days, but her sense of smell is spot-on. Newbies can immediately tell who their mothers are just by their scent.**

You can run (well, waddle) but you can't hide from all smells while pregnant, so try and avoid the ones that make you sick. If that doesn't pan out, take a tip from folks who work with stinky stuff all the time: Mask the odors by dabbing your nostrils with coconut or olive oil mixed with a drop of peppermint, eucalyptus, or any other fragrant oil that makes you happy.

 Did you hear the joke about the pregnant lady's body odor? I didn't choose to listen to it myself because I heard it stinks.

Loss Of Smell

If you're turning green at even the faintest stench, you will probably be envious of baby mamas with anosmia, which is a total loss of smell. Anosmia can be genetic or caused by a trauma to the nose, but a temporary case can also appear out of the blue when you're pregnant. It's not always entirely unwelcome—anosmia is in fact associated with a lower chance of nausea and vomiting in pregnancy. Although your usual sense of smell will likely return after giving birth, you may want to consult with your doctor if you can no longer stop and smell the roses, as there may be other possible factors such as allergies or nasal congestion at play.

Breathing Problems

Even if you're not sick or suffering from allergies, you may one day find that you're struggling mightily with nasal congestion—and chances are you have pregnancy rhinitis, which afflicts up to one-third of all mamas-to-be and is caused by the natural increase in hormones during pregnancy.

No, this doesn't mean you are being compared to a rhinoceros—*rhino* just means "nose" in Latin, and *rhinitis* refers to nasal congestion when no other respiratory issues or allergies are present. This condition can crop up anytime in pregnancy and typically involves (besides nasal congestion) sneezing, coughing, headaches, and exhaustion. As if you didn't already have enough to complain about!

Relief is available in the form of several safe home treatments that can help alleviate your symptoms (see page 86). Plus, your nose should completely clear up within a few weeks after giving birth—not that you'll be sleeping any easier then, but at least it will be because of baby and not a stopped-up schnoz.

> If you are experiencing shortness of breath, you might be having asthmatic symptoms or even an asthma attack. Tell your doctor ASAP. If left untreated, asthma can put you at risk for preterm delivery, low birth weight, and preeclampsia, which can be devastating for you and your baby (see page 4).

HOW TO ⇨ Alleviate Congestion Safely

Before you take your usual (pre-pregnancy) OTC decongestants, be sure and run them by your doctor. Some nasal sprays can even worsen your congestion if used incorrectly, and other medications have been found to be unsafe for baby, especially when taken in the first trimester.

Ugh, what's a clogged-up preggo to do? For starters, try using these alternative remedies:

- a humidifier to keep mucous membranes from drying out
- a diffuser filled with head-clearing essential oils, like peppermint or eucalyptus
- a neti pot for flushing out your nasal cavity
- saline nasal spray to soothe your nostrils
- facial steams at home to temporarily open your airways
- extra pillows to prop up your head while sleeping or lying down
- adhesive nasal strips while sleeping (because you didn't already feel sexy enough)

If your sinus problems don't let up, see your doctor to make sure there isn't an underlying issue that needs to be nipped in the bud, particularly an illness that requires a pregnancy-safe prescription.

Limiting your use of over-the-counter nasal sprays for congestion can be beneficial even when you're not pregnant. Oftentimes the more you use nasal decongestant sprays in a short period of time, the less effective they become at helping you breathe.

EYES & EARS

EYES

Vision Problems

Does it seem as if you're viewing life through one of those blurry Instagram filters lately? Do things look somehow a little different these days, for better or worse? Edema strikes again!

Fluid retention during pregnancy doesn't just produce "cankles." It can even make your eyeballs expand, altering your vision to include blurriness, clarity shifts, and even a lack of peripheral vision. This swelling can also prevent your prescription contacts from fitting properly, which can also affect your vision. If so, or if you are simply bothered by the way your contacts feel, switch to glasses and hold off on spending any money on a new prescription just yet. Your eyesight might shift even further as your pregnancy progresses and you retain more fluid, and it will hopefully go back to normal after delivery.

In other words, vision changes can simply be a normal part of pregnancy, and as long as they're not triggered by any underlying medical complications, they won't put your baby at risk. You may even find these pregnancy-induced vision changes to be a bonus, as I did: My eyesight improved so much during my second pregnancy that I was devastated when my nearsightedness came barreling back once my son was born.

Pregnant Lady #1:
"When I look in the mirror, all I see is me getting fatter. Can you give me a compliment?"
Pregnant Lady #2:
"You have perfect eyesight."

Dry Eyes

You might feel weepier while you're pregnant, but you are actually producing fewer tears now than when you're not—and this can result in dry, irritated eyes, which are especially uncomfortable if you wear contacts. Dry eyes can also worsen with a lack of sleep.

Blinded by the light? You're not imagining things. Pregnancy can make your eyes more sensitive to brightness, particularly from the sun, so wear sunglasses when you're outside (or even in an especially sunny spot inside) to avoid discomfort.

Your scratchy eyes will generally go back to normal by the time your baby is six months old, but until then you can use artificial tears for soothing relief; make sure they are safe for contacts if you wear those. Wearing glasses instead of contact lenses can also help. If the dryness worsens, your doctor may be able to prescribe safe (and super-soothing!) prescription drops or eye ointments.

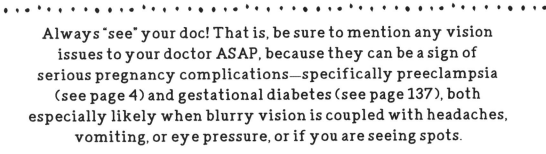

Always "see" your doc! That is, be sure to mention any vision issues to your doctor ASAP, because they can be a sign of serious pregnancy complications—specifically preeclampsia (see page 4) and gestational diabetes (see page 137), both especially likely when blurry vision is coupled with headaches, vomiting, or eye pressure, or if you are seeing spots.

Watery Eyes

As odd as it sounds, watery eyes can be symptomatic of dry eye (yes, really); they can also be due to allergies. Either way, you are not imagining things if it seems like you're tearing up more than usual—and for no other apparent reason.

If your eyes are sensitive, eye makeup can make things even worse. Ditch the liner and mascara for a while to see if that helps.

EARS

Burning Ears

Out of nowhere, say while driving your car, your ears feel like they're on fire and you swear there's smoke spilling out both sides of your head just like in the cartoons. You glance in the rearview mirror and, sure enough, your ears (or maybe just one ear) are (is) bright red.

If that sounds at all familiar, it wasn't just your imagination on overdrive. Rather, this pregnancy side effect is like a hot flash—or, better yet, a power surge—that causes the blood to rush into your outer ears (see more about hot flashes on page 18). Other than putting your lobes on ice, this surreal symptom just needs to be waited out.

> Did you hear about the deaf OB-GYN? She could read lips!

Hearing Loss

Just when you thought you'd heard it all, so to speak, your sense of hearing might drop off a bit during pregnancy, thanks to water and salt retention. Never *fear*: Your hearing will almost always pick back up after giving birth—just in time to hear baby's cries and coos.

Earwax

Weirdly enough, earwax is yet another of the bodily secretions that many women say increases during pregnancy. This excess wax may contribute to other pregnancy-related ear problems, such as hearing loss (see page 90) and tinnitus (see page 92). You may also experience a blockage from too much earwax, or because you inadvertently pushed the wax into your ears when cleaning them out with a cotton swab—always a big no-no. Instead, if your mucked-up ears are driving you mad, head to your doctor's office for a professional (and perfectly safe) ear cleaning. Besides potentially alleviating the discomfort, this quick procedure feels really (and strangely) good.

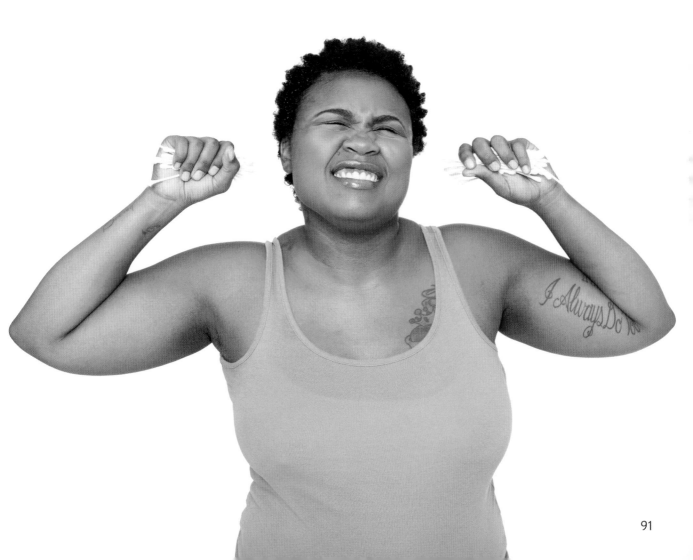

Ear Pain or Swelling

If you feel any pain or notice swelling in your ears, let your doctor know ASAP. Pregnancy rhinitis (see page 85), which causes nasal stuffiness, postnasal drip, and congestion, can lead to fluid retention in the middle ear and can easily turn into a middle-ear infection. It is also possible for an infection from the nose to spread to the middle ear through the Eustachian tube. The sooner you catch these conditions, the easier it will be to treat them.

Ringing Ears (Tinnitus)

The most common ear issue in pregnancy is tinnitus, which involves the disconcerting sensation of hearing whizzing, ringing, buzzing, sizzling, or similar phantom noises. Up to one-quarter of pregnant women suffer from this problem, which can be a sign of preeclampsia (see page 4) or another serious issue, but most often will prove to be yet another annoying thorn in your pregnancy side.

Your growing baby can actually hear you! Starting in the third trimester, babies learn how to recognize words, music, and sounds. One study discovered that mothers who often watched a soap opera while pregnant had babies that recognized the show's theme song.

HANDS & FEET

HANDS

Caught Red-handed?

Up to one-third of pregnant women deal with palmar erythema, a sensation of warmth coupled with redness on the hands that may appear to be an inflammatory condition or a friction-caused rash. It can affect one or both hands, and sometimes only a few fingers.

Occasionally, a similar affliction called plantar erythema can occur on the soles of the feet—usually the entirety of both soles, if at all.

In general, palmar erythema is known to be a symptom of liver problems, lupus, and rheumatoid arthritis, but in a mom-to-be, it is simply a common pregnancy side effect. It won't harm you or your baby and should disappear after delivery.

Tingling Hands or Wrists

As soon as your pregnancy became the talk of your town, everyone was probably quick to warn you about heartburn and constipation. But they may have forgotten to mention the pins-and-needles sensation that's now making your hands feel as clumsy and uncomfortable as your other bodily parts. If the tingling in your hands and wrists doesn't go away after a couple of shake-shake-shakes, it's probably more than just the upshot of sleeping the wrong way last night. While several nonpregnancy-related causes exist, it's most likely a (fingers crossed!) temporary case of carpal tunnel syndrome (CTS) brought on by pregnancy.

Located in the wrist, the carpal tunnel acts as a passageway for several important nerves and tendons (notably the median nerve) that are to thank for your pre-pregnancy ability to feel and move most of your fingers. Unfortunately, swelling during pregnancy also affects your wrists, pinching the tunnel and nerves located there. While the pain or numbness this causes might seem scary at first, it's in fact fairly common—nearly two-thirds of pregnant women may experience these sensations.

Although your symptoms will likely go away after you give birth, there are many ways to help you manage them until your due date. Many of the activities we do in our daily lives put pressure on the nerves and consequently make CTS worse. Repeated movements such as typing, knitting, or playing instruments aggravate the problem, so although you might be tired of hearing it by now, the best solution is to frequently give your wrists a rest.

Admittedly, making like the Sphinx and lying with your wrists completely motionless isn't everyone's cup of tea. If you're dead set on finishing that cross-stitch project to warmly welcome the long-awaited addition to your family, or can't give up certain activities because of your work, be sure to build in plenty of breaks.

Using a wrist brace or splint to make sure your wrist stays in the correct position, and pressure free, may also help. Wearing the splint to bed will give you the most benefit for your buck. Symptoms tend to get worse at night, and with all the tossing and turning, who knows how you're bending your wrists?

Under the right circumstances, some bending can be useful. Wrist exercises such as shaking your hands vigorously, doing finger push-ups, and CTS-specific stretches like pressing your hands together in prayer position can all ease and even help prevent carpal tunnel syndrome.

Even though CTS is most likely behind the tingling pain, it's a good idea to tell your doctor just in case there may be another culprit, including anemia (see page 128), a vitamin B12 deficiency, or hypothyroidism. If it turns out that your numbness is caused by anemia, your doctor might recommend taking an iron supplement or eating more iron-rich foods, including red meat, beans, and spinach. Similarly, he may suggest upping your folic acid intake for a vitamin B12 deficiency. Avoid the urge to self-diagnose and make any intense changes to your diet or buy unapproved vitamins from the drugstore. Talk to your doctor first.

De Quervain's Tenosynovitis

Because it often shows up in new mothers, and involves the tendons in the thumb side of the wrist, de Quervain's tenosynovitis (dih-kwer-VAINS ten-oh-sine-oh-VIE-tis) has

been given a much easier-to-remember (and-to-pronounce) nickname: "mommy thumb." But this painful condition can crop up in pregnant women, too.

For new moms, de Quervain's is often related to the many gripping movements that are part and parcel of caring for their newborns, including nursing and lifting them throughout the day and night. In pregnancy, even the most mundane activities can trigger the condition, making it easy

Struggling with itchy hands and feet? Check out the skin section on page 8 for more information on possible causes, including intrahepatic cholestasis of pregnancy (ICP) or dyshidrotic eczema.

to mistake it for carpal tunnel syndrome (see pages 94–5). Have your doctor diagnose it for you (or refer you to a specialist) so you can choose the appropriate support brace that will help alleviate your particular pain.

NAILS

Nails That Separate

One or more of your nails might start separating from the end of its nail bed in what is called onycholysis. If the area where the nail is separating starts looking yellow and scaly, you may have subungual hyperkeratosis, as do around 4 percent of pregnant women. There's a chance onycholysis and subungual hyperkeratosis could be caused by a fungus or an infection, so pay a visit to the doctor to nail down a diagnosis.

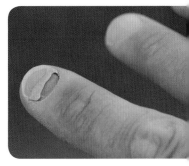

Brittle Nails

It's not just a sleight of hand: Your nails may, indeed, be growing faster. They may even be growing so fast that they don't have time to strengthen and instead just remain weak—and more prone to tearing or breaking. Nearly 10 percent of pregnant women deal with especially brittle, splitting nails, a condition that goes by the daunting name of onychoschizia.

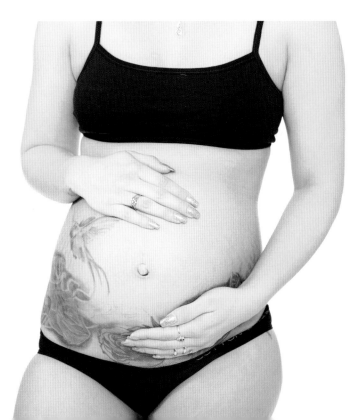

Ingrown Toenails

You've gone your entire life without an ingrown toenail, yet suddenly, now that you're knocked up, your feet are all jacked up. Coincidence? Absolutely not! Even though it

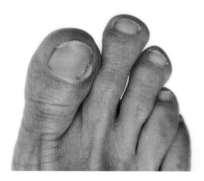

seems that no other pregnancy book talks about this issue, it is fairly common for a woman to get at least one ingrown toenail during pregnancy—and it is often her first time dealing with one.

Formally known as onychocryptosis, an ingrown toenail is one that seems to deliberately dig down into the sides or corners of the surrounding tissue, resulting in swelling, pain, and redness. If infected, you may also see bleeding or pus.

What makes ingrown toenails so likely in pregnancy? For starters, you're producing an excess of foot sweat that softens the nail and makes it more likely to split and puncture the surrounding skin. Also, pregnancy-related swelling often causes shoes and socks to fit more snugly; the swelling then frequently descends to the fingers and toes, causing extra pressure around the nail tissue. These changes create a hotbed for an ingrown nail to develop.

The best way to stave off ingrown toenails is by wearing socks and shoes that have plenty of room in the toe area. And contrary to what you might think, getting frequent pedicures might actually be promoting—rather than solving—the problem! Whoever is cutting your nails should make sure to

> If your nails develop horizontal ridges, you could have "Beau's lines," a.k.a. transverse grooving. These harmless lines appear when your body slows down the production of nail cells, which sometimes happens in pregnancy.

- file or cut your nails straight across, without tapering or rounding off the nail corners;
- avoid cutting your nails without soaking them in water first;
- and never cut your nails too short.

If you do end up with an ingrown nail (with all due sympathy), take steps to keep it from becoming infected. A podiatrist should be your first stop if you have diabetes, nerve damage, or a circulatory issue, or if the pain or swelling is spreading beyond your nail—do not attempt to treat this yourself in these circumstances.

If you don't have any of the above concerns, try to get your ingrown nail under control by wearing comfortable shoes (preferably open-toed), and by soaking the affected digit in warm water a few times a day, with or without Epsom salts. If this doesn't help, and the pain is getting worse—or if you think it's infected because of blood or pus—see your doctor, who may be able to remove the embedded nail section and prescribe medications to ease the pain and other symptoms.

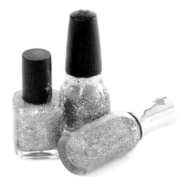

Up to one-quarter of pregnant women report the appearance of white spots on their nails. Although these innocuous specks are usually caused by an injury, they seem to appear in pregnancy for no reason.

FEET

Permanent Foot Growth

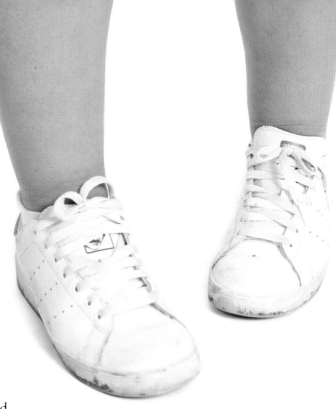

Love your Jimmy Choos? Well, be prepared to kiss them goodbye, because they just might not fit after your pregnancy—and no amount of pleading to the shoe gods will help one bit. Alas, permanent foot growth is one of many modifications your body will undergo during pregnancy. All your extra weight, combined with your old friend relaxin, causes the ligaments in your tired dogs to loosen and stretch and the arch in your feet to flatten a bit, resulting in the need for a shoe size that's bigger in length (typically around ten millimeters, or up one size) and width.

Despite what you may be thinking, you're not going to become the next Big Foot. Subsequent pregnancies don't seem to have the same effect, so no matter how many children you have, your feet probably won't grow after your first is born—and you and your fave new shoes can strut happily ever after!

While ballet slippers and flip-flops are better than high heels, flats and flops lack the support a healthy pregnant foot needs to be strong and stable. If you want to help your feet (and back), choose sensible, well-fitting shoes with good arch and ankle support. In other words, for the next nine months put form and function above fashion.

Calluses and Corns

The stress that pregnancy puts on your feet can lead to some quite uncomfortable (and unseemly in sandal season) developments. Calluses develop when the skin of your swollen feet rubs against too-tight shoes, resulting in a thickening of the skin that may cause those shoes to fit even worse than before. Corns are hard, thick bumps of skin that usually grow, as a protective response to some ill-fitting shoes, over a bone in certain areas of your feet.

When and if these growths happen to you (or better yet, before they happen), it's time to wear more comfortable shoes or run the risk of making the problem worse. Have your partner or a professional remove calluses with a pumice stone; if the growths are particularly troubling, see a podiatrist. For corns, which can be much more painful than calluses, keep your feet well moisturized, rubbing your favorite lotion or coconut oil onto your heels and other dry areas at least once per day—more if you have the time and someone to apply it.

After baby is born, your calluses and corns may start to recede, and even if they don't, you will no longer have a baby bump to keep you from tending to these sore spots yourself.

> Socks that are too tight, socks that bunch up because they are too loose, or even a weirdly placed sock seam can rub your feet the wrong way and cause the same kinds of foot problems as a poorly fitting shoe.

 A new mom went to her podiatrist to have a corn removed. After the procedure, she asked whether she needed a follow-up appointment. The doctor replied, "No, but if you have any problems, please callus back."

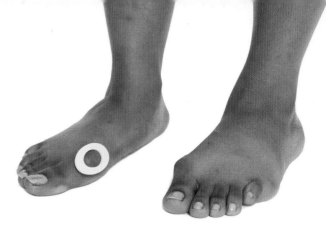

Bunions

If you never had bunions prior to becoming pregnant, guess what? You got it—or at least you're likely to get one of these annoyances now that you are a mama-to-be. And if you already have one, it can take a turn for the worse.

Bunions appear as large bumps on the inside of the foot at the base of your big toe and are thanks to your loosening pregnancy ligaments, which are no longer doing their job of holding the bones of your feet together as effectively as they used to—hence, the foot can become disfigured. Although not dangerous, bunions are no fun-ions. They can be painful as well as permanent—and therefore must be treated by a podiatrist, sometimes with surgery.

Trading in stilettos for some admittedly less sexy footwear for the next few months is the smart thing to do, right? Still, one-third of tortured pregnant soles (er, souls) indicated in a recent survey that they were still wearing pumps throughout their pregnancy.

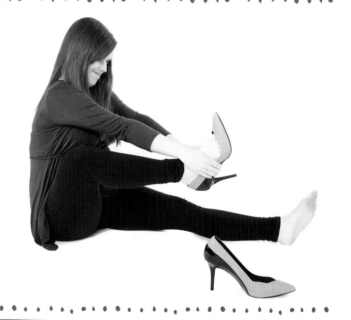

TEETH, MOUTH & THROAT

⋙ Put this book down and make an appointment with your dentist ASAP! Studies show that taking care of your teeth during pregnancy not only can improve your health and self-esteem, but also can potentially decrease the risk of preterm and low-birth-weight deliveries. Your good dental hygiene may even reduce the incidence of future childhood tooth decay for baby.

Drooling: Not Just For Babies!

Have you swallowed more than the usual amount of saliva lately? Do you find yourself spitting often, only to have the saliva build right back up again? Welcome to ptyalism gravidarum, which can begin before you even miss your first period and last throughout the first trimester—or, for a few unlucky women, until delivery. This saliva spout can happen while you are awake or asleep, and it tends to spoil the taste and experience of eating and life in general.

Because no one has identified the precise cause of pregnancy ptyalism, it can be difficult to come up with a treatment plan. If you are experiencing heartburn, nausea, and/or vomiting (ptyalism is commonly seen in hyperemesis gravidarum sufferers; see page 122), that may be a clue. The salivary glands could be irritated by a surplus of stomach acids, so you can try and ease those symptoms.

Otherwise, you'll just have to go with the overflow. Some women carry around cups (or gobs of tissue) to spit into; keep a cup on the bedside table, too, for nocturnal spurts.

Dry Mouth

At the other end of the spittle spectrum is sandpaper mouth—lack of saliva, officially called xerostomia, is also common in pregnancy. Not only is it unpleasant, but dry mouth can also cause complications in your oral health, including mouth sores and infections (page 115), gum disease, chewing problems, and tooth decay. Turns out that bacteria have an easier time adhering to tissues that are dry rather than moist, especially when there's not enough saliva to wash away the food particles that can remain on your teeth and lead to decay.

Here are some suggestions for wetting your whistle:

- drink more water or suck on chips of ice (but fluid intake alone may not solve the problem completely)
- chew sugarless gum or suck on sugar-free candies to help stimulate saliva
- use mouthwashes that are specifically designed to moisten oral tissue (or use OTC saliva substitutes)—just make sure to buy one that is completely natural and free of sugar and alcohol to avoid making your problem worse
- limit your caffeine intake (which you should be doing anyway), as it can make your mouth even drier

As always, you should be brushing twice a day for optimum oral health, but this is especially important when you suffer from dry mouth, as is brushing before bed because dry mouth often worsens at night. For this reason, you may also want to run a humidifier while you sleep to help to relieve symptoms.

Dry mouth can be more than just irritating—it can also be a symptom of anemia (page 128) and gestational diabetes (page 137), so be sure to tell your doctor about your complaints, even if you've been cleared for these medical issues.

Snoring more now that you're pregnant? Mouth breathing while sleeping can be an unexpected cause of dry mouth in the morning.

Voice Variations

Say it isn't so! Scientific evidence has proven that anatomic, metabolic, and physiologic changes during pregnancy can influence the characteristics and quality of your voice. Here are some reasons why you might be having a pregnancy-related voice change:

- **Upswing in hormones.** The vast increase in estrogen and progesterone levels in the body can affect the thickness of the vocal cords, resulting in a change in the pitch of your voice.
- **Rise in body fluid levels.** During pregnancy, your blood volume increases (by 50 percent!), which accounts for a full six pounds of your weight gain. When this excess fluid concentrates near the vocal cords, it causes them to vibrate at a different rate—and hence to lower the pitch of your voice.
- **Vocal cord swelling.** The vocal cords can swell up and become heavier while you are pregnant, thereby preventing you from singing in your normal range—often this means no more high notes. Avoid straining to hit those high notes, too; you can tear your fragile arteries and veins (see below) or even the vocal cords themselves. (In other words, no singin' in the pain!)
- **Lowered nasal resonance.** Your nasal cavities can also swell during pregnancy, making breathing through your nose difficult, and creating a decline in nasal (and sinus) resonance such that your voice becomes deeper and husky sounding. Consider it a pregnancy perk!
- **Dilation of arteries and veins.** While you are pregnant, the arteries and veins will enlarge throughout your body, including those in the area of your vocal cords, leaving them more susceptible to rupturing and tearing—especially if you strain your voice. This situation can also cause a deepening of your voice.
- **Decreased lung capacity.** Pregnancy is a time in which it is often hard to breathe, mostly because the growing fetus inside the uterus will push on your diaphragm, thereby decreasing the air capacity of your lungs. This produces a decline in voice endurance and the ability to sing along with vocal cord fatigue.
- **Increase in laryngopharyngeal reflux.** While you are pregnant, the valve that keeps stomach acid out of your esophagus and away from your vocal cords is not as strong;

as a result, your vocal cords can become so irritated by the exposure to acid that your voice can crack and you can also experience a sore throat.

- **Posture changes.** Because your center of gravity shifts and your posture is not the same during pregnancy, your vocal cords are not getting the same support when you talk or sing. In fact, singing in the third trimester can be very difficult.

Talk to your doctor if you experience pain whenever you talk or try to sing, if there is a sudden change in your singing or speaking voice (especially after you cough or sneeze), or if you lose your voice at any point during pregnancy. While none of these occurrences will affect your baby, they might affect your singing career—but only temporarily. You should be speaking and singing in your old voice after baby is born—just in time for fairy tales and lullabies.

What do you call a bad joke about a pregnant woman's weird tongue issues? Tasteless!

Do-re-mi-fa-so-la-preg-oh-NO!

Swollen Lips

If you've ever wondered what your face would look like if you enhanced your natural pout with lip injections, you're in luck—pregnancy just might afford you a free trial. In fact, many women find themselves being asked if they've gotten their lips plumped up well before they're ready to announce their pregnancy. Talk about a subtle, yet sexy, giveaway!

Before you get too carried away with getting a complimentary "celeb look," there may be a catch: Because the surrounding skin is being stretched beyond its normal limits, your swollen lips might be accompanied by throbbing, chapping, and cracking, especially in the susceptible corners of your mouth.

Your perkier pecker should be relatively constant during pregnancy. Talk to your doctor if the swelling ebbs and flows, and especially if you have pain or trouble breathing—this could be a sign that the swelling is related to a severe allergic reaction (which will require an antihistamine) or a dental issue. Pay special attention to an increase in these symptoms if they happen, along with the swelling in your lips, when you eat or drink.

In general, however, swelling is just a natural, normal part of pregnancy—and this time, it happens in a place many people pay to puff. If you aren't a fan of the fullness, try placing cold compresses on your lips to reduce the swelling: As often as you please, wet a washcloth with cold water, wring it out, and fold or roll it up, then place it across your mouth, preferably while lying down. (Note: You can do the same thing, at the same time, to soothe your tired eyes—for the ultimate in cool comfort.) Even if this doesn't alleviate your particular kind of swelling, it will still feel good! Be sure to protect your kisser from cracked and chapped lips by frequently applying a high-quality lip balm or even coconut oil (see page 110 for more on crusty kissers).

If there's no underlying cause for the mysterious plumping other than pregnancy, you can expect your lips to go back to normal within weeks of giving birth. If they don't, then you should keep mentioning it to your doctor and get a second (or third) opinion until someone takes your concerns seriously.

Whatever caused the swelling, there's a small chance that the resulting stretching will lead to a higher risk of developing perioral wrinkles (a.k.a. "mouth lines"), which can cause lipsticks to bleed. If this matters to you, double down your efforts to stay hydrated and moisturized, and be diligent about your skin regime to retain as much elasticity as possible.

Baby Blue . . . Lips?

Emotional baby blues are one thing to keep an eye out for (see page 178 for more on pre-natal depression)—and blue lips in pregnancy are another. Depending on your natural skin and lip hues, a new blue or purple tint to your pucker can signify a variety of pregnancy complications, some more problematic than others. A "cool" change in lip color during pregnancy could merely be a hormonal side effect, but call your doctor just in case, because your bluish or purplish lips could also suggest:

- **Iron deficiency (anemia).** Blue lips can be a symptom (see page 128 for more on this).
- **Circulation and breathing problems.** Poor circulation and low oxygen levels are possible reasons behind blue- or purple-tinged lips. If, along with your new hue, you have any heart-related ailments in your family history, or if you are having problems breathing or are asthmatic—or simply don't feel well—call your doctor and report your symptoms ASAP.
- **Pneumonia or other lung conditions, a blood clot, or a heart problem.** These and other serious issues can also cause bluish lips; if any of them might be a concern, stop reading this book and call your doctor ASAP.

It's not just your lips that can look like you've stayed too long in the blueberry bushes. A blue hue in your gums, around your eyes, and in your fingernail and toenail beds can point to the same concerns, so keep an eye on all these body parts—and once your ever-growing belly prevents you from seeing your toes, put that color-check on your part-ner's ever-growing to-do-for-you list!

Chapped & Cracked Lips

One of the first signs that you are pregnant is sometimes having chapped lips. (Um, congrats!) Chapped and cracked lips are not just unattractive and often painful; they can also serve as a vehicle for a bacterial infection to pass through your bloodstream to the baby. Common causes include mouth breathing, dehydration, and an infection called angular cheilitis (see below).

During pregnancy, the nasal mucosa (the membranes lining the nasal cavity) can become so engorged that it is difficult to breathe through your nose (see page 85 for more on pregnancy rhinitis). All that breathing through your mouth ends up drying your lips out and makes them susceptible to chapping. Saline nasal drops might help to clear your nose so you no longer have to breathe through your mouth. Steer clear of medicinal nasal sprays, however, unless approved by your doctor, in case the one in your medicine cabinet is not cleared for pregnancy (see page 86 for more on this).

If mouth breathing is not to blame, your problem might be dehydration. For the fifty-first time, drink more water!

Angular Cheilitis

Pregnant women can get an infection and inflammation around the corners of the mouth called angular cheilitis. Usually this happens because of increased stress in pregnancy as well as iron and vitamin deficiencies (especially B vitamins) and other nutritional insufficiencies.

Angular cheilitis is more common during the first trimester, when morning sickness is at its worst. Signs of this condition include chapped and flaky skin and also the appearance of painful sores that may develop. Talk to your doctor to rule out anything more serious than just plain ol' boring chapped lips—and keep a steady supply of your favorite balm on hand for soothing relief.

Geographic Tongue Twisters

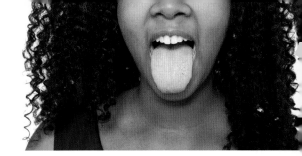

Map got your tongue? Do the top and sides of your tongue have patches of various shapes, colors, and sizes, each with a light-colored or whitish border? If so, you may very well have an odd-sounding condition called geographic tongue, which is not at all odd to have in pregnancy. To put it as simply as possible, while your tongue is normally covered with papillae, tiny bumps that give the tongue its rough texture (and which are covered in even tinier taste buds), sometimes those tiny bumps disappear in spots—creating those irregular patches, which can move and change quickly over several days or weeks.

It's not clear why certain people lose their papillae. Sometimes the condition runs in families and may be a matter of genetics; it's also seen in people who have a tongue fissure or who suffer from psoriasis (page 21). Studies have shown a possible link involving increased hormone levels during pregnancy, too. Lesions may worsen with increased stress, after eating spicy and acidic foods, and when using teeth-whitening toothpaste.

Whatever the cause, geographic tongue is completely harmless. It is a benign tongue condition that isn't caused by an infection and won't lead to cancer. Fortunately, it only produces tongue sensitivity in about 10 percent of cases, and most people do not even realize anything is amiss until a dentist or doctor mentions it during an examination.

Generally, geographic tongue lasts the entire pregnancy and in some instances for a short while after delivery. In the meantime, you'll just have to plant your tongue firmly in your cheek (in a manner of speaking).

As you gain pregnancy weight, so might your tongue. This increase in size may be behind your nocturnal tossing and turning, as a fatter tongue is more likely to block your airway, causing sleep disorders like sleep apnea (page 147). Mention any noticeable growth spurt to your doctor.

Oral Thrush

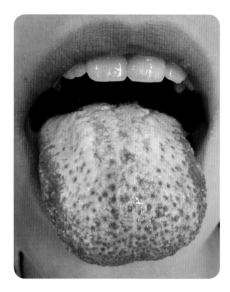

Oral thrush is basically a yeast infection in your mouth. Now that you've died a little, you may take comfort in knowing that this development is all too common in pregnancy, when your immune system lacks the ability to fight off yeast organisms that occur naturally in the mouth—and which can lead to a buildup of yeast and, consequently, oral thrush. (Are you sitting down? Besides the tongue, thrush can develop on the genitals as well as on the nipples of mothers who are breastfeeding a baby who has thrush.)

The main symptom of oral thrush is whitish or yellowish lesions or patches that often appear as a thick film on the tongue (and sometimes elsewhere in the mouth). Those with oral thrush may experience dry mouth and a decreased sense of taste, and in the severest of cases, cracking or soreness that can lead to bleeding spots and difficulty eating certain foods.

Swallow your pride (ha!) and alert your doctor, who can help you manage the condition. You can also treat the infection with saltwater rinses and twice-daily brushing and flossing, and by steering clear of alcohol-based mouthwashes, which can make the mouth even more prone to thrush and other disorders. After baby is born, your immune system will normalize and the oral thrush will likely go away.

Tonsil Stones

Along with growing your baby, you might be growing "tonsilloliths," officially known as tonsil stones. These hard, calcified stones collect in the crevices of the tonsils and make you feel like there is something stuck in the back of your throat. They can also cause a sore throat and coughing. Tonsil stones are formed in the same way in which a pearl is produced—that is, if a pearl was made from a gross mixture of food particles, bacteria, and white blood cells that gives your breath a sulfuric foulness.

Tonsil stones often dislodge and disappear on their own, but if they're bothering you, talk to your doctor. Avoid doing what others have done—do not try to dislodge them with chopsticks or straws (or even a cotton swab, which can work, but not on your own). Tonsils are delicate and can be easily damaged.

There's nothing dangerous about tonsil stones, but they might stick around after baby is born. Sometimes, the only relief is to have your tonsils removed so the stones have no place to grow, but because your tonsils serve a protective purpose, this route is not always recommended.

Hiccups

During pregnancy, hiccups are bound to happen—in life, and also in your throat. Now that you have a baby on board, you're taking in 30 to 40 percent more air per breath than when you weren't pregnant, and for good reason: Your body, and the baby's body, need extra oxygen to support increased cellular function. Unfortunately, all that excess air can (and probably will) land in your stomach, triggering your diaphragm to spasm, and the hiccups to commence.

That's just one scenario. There are actually more than one hundred known causes of hiccups, yet no sure way to prevent them. Fortunately, most hiccups will stop on their own, though there have been cases where a serious bout lasted for more than forty-eight hours—and which would mandate a trip to the doctor's office to prevent the persistent hiccups from interfering with normal eating and sleeping patterns.

"Treatment" is the same as for nonpregnancy hiccups: Take deep breaths, eat more slowly, and drink small sips of water with each bite. And be prepared for friends and family (and anyone else within earshot) to share their very own time-tested tips and tricks for you to try, too.

Bleeding Gums (Gingivitis)

Bleeding gums are a side effect of pregnancy gingivitis, an inflammation of the gums caused by an increase in plaque, the nasty film of bacteria that coats the teeth and gums. Gingivitis affects up to 70 percent of pregnant women, and besides causing other oral hygiene problems such as bad breath, loosened teeth, and tooth decay, it can progress into a more severe form of gum disease called periodontitis, which some studies have shown increases the chance of preterm birth.

See your dentist at least once during your pregnancy for a routine cleaning and to have your teeth and gums examined. If you are found to have pregnancy gingivitis (or perhaps you had it before you conceived), your dentist can lay out a plan of action to keep the inflammation in check.

Bad Breath

Aside from gingivitis (see above), there are many other reasons your pregnancy reeks—breathwise, that is. Tonsil stones (page 112), dry mouth (page 105), and dehydration (page 126) are other possible causes of bad breath, as is frequent vomiting (page 120), when odors from partially digested food and stomach acid can linger. Make sure to schedule a dental checkup during pregnancy, as your dentist will be able to offer suggestions to safely keep bad breath at bay.

Pregnancy Granuloma

Are your gums starring in their own horror flick of late? Up to 10 percent of women deal with painful, but totally benign, purple or red tumors (a.k.a. granuloma) that crop up in the mouth, but most commonly along the gumline. They can be anywhere from a few millimeters to a few inches in diameter and might interfere with chewing and drinking; if irritated, they can bleed and turn into either an open or crusted-over sore, neither result being pleasant.

Thought to be related to increased hormone production, granuloma cannot be prevented or treated, but your dentist can help you get through this bizarre pregnancy complication. And while you can certainly ask to have them removed during pregnancy, the tumors often come back; they also usually shrink down and go away after giving birth, so your best bet might be to simply grin and bear them.

Mouth Sores

Mouth sores, also called canker or cold sores, are extremely common in pregnancy and can pop up anywhere, including the tongue, gums, cheek lining, palate, and inner lips. They usually look like blisters at first; if they burst, you're left with shallow ulcers that can sting like mad, make it painful to talk or eat, and even lead to bad breath.

In general, mouth sores can be caused by taking certain medications or accidentally biting your inner cheek. Some possible reasons they are more common in pregnancy include vitamin deficiencies, increased stress, and lowered immunity.

It is more difficult to treat mouth sores during pregnancy because many of the topical medications are not safe for your baby. Talk to your doctor about possible options, including lidocaine mouthwashes and all-natural treatments. Other basic remedies for mouth sores in pregnancy include eating a bland diet, gargling with salt water, and trying to reduce your stress level (as if).

Should you be unlucky enough to suffer a mouth sore during your pregnancy, alert your dentist or doctor to rule out an underlying condition or infection. Otherwise, mouth sores usually clear up soon after you deliver.

After a male cardinalfish courts a female, he carries the fertilized eggs in his mouth, and is unable to eat for weeks until they hatch.

Loose Teeth

Along with the bones and ligaments in the rest of your body, those that support your teeth are also affected by pregnancy, meaning you may find that your previously sturdy molars are now wiggling like they did in elementary school. Good news: If there is no underlying tooth decay or gum disease, your chompers will return to their rock-steady state once baby is born. But rather than being caused by decay or gum disease, this unsettling phenomenon is due to (no surprise!) hormonal changes. Your dentist will be able to tell the difference between pregnancy-related loose teeth and more serious concerns.

Painful Teeth

Tooth erosion and weakened enamel can be painful, especially if you also have tooth decay. One theory holds that pregnant women are more likely to have this problem because they eat more decay-causing sweets (sure, blame the victim!). Generally, however, these dental difficulties are more often found in women suffering from nausea and vomiting during pregnancy: The stomach acid that comes up when you vomit eats away at the enamel surface that usually protects the teeth from decay and, consequently, makes your teeth more prone to cavities (see page 120 for more on vomiting).

Although brushing your teeth twice a day is essential to maintaining healthy teeth, you should not brush your teeth immediately after a bout of vomiting—brushing now will further exacerbate the potential damage. Instead, after vomiting, rinse your mouth out with an acid-neutralizing solution made by mixing a teaspoon of baking soda with a cup of water.

If you are experiencing frequent vomiting, or if you gag at the sight of a toothbrush, see page 117 for toothbrush alternatives that are safer for your sensitive gums and teeth.

HOW TO ⇨ Brush Your Teeth Without a Toothbrush

The old wives' tale, "Gain a Child, Lose a Tooth," is indeed rooted in reality. For many pregnant women, the mere feel of a toothbrush on their tongue is enough to make them heave. You can't just give oral hygiene the brush-off, however; you still need to clean away plaque to prevent tooth decay and gingivitis (see page 114). So what's a toothbrush-hating gal to do?

When you are suffering from near-constant nausea (as discussed on page 120), or are dealing with harmless but painful mouth sores (see page 115) or aching teeth (see page 116), the toothbrush can seem more like a weapon of mass destruction than of the cavity-and-crown-prevention tool it is designed to be. And let's be wide open (or open wide!): It's much easier to skip brushing altogether and let pregnancy wreak havoc on your pearly whites than to deal with all the pain and puking. I'll spare you the lectures on the importance of brushing your teeth. Instead, here's a palatable toothbrush alternative that will help keep you kiss-ably fresh and filling free until the big day.

What You'll Need:
- a washcloth (the small ones for babies work great, and you can reuse them for your own tiny tot)
- toothpaste if you can stomach it, baking soda if you cannot
- a cup (to rinse your mouth out)

Step 1)   Wet the washcloth in whatever temperature of water won't make you hurl.

Step 2)   Wrap it around your pointer finger (like a mini ghost costume) and add the toothpaste or baking soda.

Step 3)   Use your finger like a toothbrush to clean each individual tooth with a rubbing, circular motion. Start with your front top teeth (less likely to induce gagging) and work your way toward the top back teeth on either side, giving yourself breaks as necessary.

Step 4)   Rinse the washcloth and reapply toothpaste (if using) and clean the bottom teeth, again starting in the front and working your way back.

Step 5)   Rinse the washcloth and use it to massage your gums and wipe your tongue.

Step 6)   Fill your cup with water and rinse your mouth out.

Alternatively, you can buy a baby toothbrush (the kind you wear like a finger puppet) and try using that if you aren't revolted by the plastic feel.

TMJ & Bite Changes

Pregnancy can bite sometimes—never more so than when you have jaw pain. After all, your sleep is disrupted, your hormones are raging, and your immunity is weakened. Plus your morning-sickness vomiting may be putting pressure on, or overextending, your neck and jaw, and your bite might even change. Due to all the stress and strain of pregnancy, you may also be grinding your teeth as you sleep, without even realizing it.

Add up all these elements and—ta-da!—you are a perfect candidate for temporomandibular joint disorder (TMJ), or inflammation of the joint that moves your jawbone (also called TMJ). You'll know you have it if you have pain and/or stiffness in your jaw along with a clicking sensation when you open and close your mouth; headaches are another symptom. And if you had a TMJ disorder prior to becoming pregnant, it is likely to flare up now that you are.

There is some evidence that temporomandibular disorders (TMD), including TMJ, are related to increased estrogen and progesterone levels during our reproductive years—a whopping 80 percent of those treated for TMJ are women, and mostly women between the ages of twenty and forty.

Besides maintaining proper oral hygiene, you need to de-stress your life as much as possible to help keep your jaw relaxed (and to prevent grinding your teeth, if you're prone to this). Meditation, yoga, gentle exercise—whatever it takes to reduce your anxiety. It's also a good idea to talk to your dentist, who will be able to assess the specific sources of your problems and offer solutions (including wearing a nighttime mouth guard to maintain a healthy bite, if warranted).

FOOD & NUTRITION

What goes in (and comes out of) your mouth during pregnancy can be cause for concern on many fronts. There's the fear that what you eat or drink might either hurt the baby or your chances of ever fitting back into your favorite jeans. Also, pregnancy symptoms might be making it difficult for you to eat certain things—or anything at all. In other words, a mom-to-be's meal is never just a meal—it's a potential minefield.

Morning Sickness All Day Long

Whoever coined the term "morning sickness" obviously never experienced it firsthand—this condition can, and will, strike any time of day or night. At any rate, this is the by-now widely accepted nickname for nausea and vomiting in pregnancy, also known as NVP (proving that everything has an acronym in pregnancy!). And in case you aren't up on the difference between the two: Nausea is the awful feeling that is often, but not always, the prelude to a bout of vomiting, which is when you expel (or "throw up") the contents of your stomach—and is just the absolute worst.

While the last thing you want to be is an MVP of NVP, chances are you will be, as nausea/vomiting is the most common side effect of pregnancy, affecting a whopping 85 percent of preggos. For most women, the symptoms subside in the second trimester; 20 percent of women, however, have them throughout their entire pregnancy—either as nausea alone or combined with vomiting. When the sickness is severe, it's known as hyperemesis gravidarum (see page 122).

Physically, NVP is a nightmare, because throwing up all that acid from your stomach often leaves you with a sore throat while also eroding the protective enamel surface on your teeth. As discussed on page 116, and contrary to what you may think, you should not brush

Only humans experience nausea and vomiting in pregnancy. No other mammal experiences these symptoms! Researchers think that we might vomit as a matter of protection because our diet is more varied than those of other living beings, meaning there are more opportunities to eat or drink something that might harm the fetus.

your teeth after every vomit; this action can promote further damage to your teeth (you'd literally be scrubbing the gastric acid into the enamel). Instead, rinse your mouth out with either plain water or a mixture of baking soda and water, and wait at least thirty minutes after your last vomit before breaking out the toothbrush (or the toothbrush alternative described on page 117 if your toothbrush makes you even more nauseated).

NVP is emotionally exhausting, too. When it strikes, even the strongest, fittest of women become discombobulated and often lose the will to do anything other than hover by a trash can or bathroom, hoping for a break that usually comes only in the form of more vomiting. Because of this infuriating infirmity, NVP can also exhaust your bank account: Morning sickness forces many pregnant women to miss work (bye-bye extra sick days for maternity leave) or, because cooking odors can trigger a bout of vomiting, to spend an inordinate amount of money on takeout or restaurant tabs.

If this sounds like you, activate your support system, and let your friends and family (and your boss if you have one) know that you're not flaking out—you're just temporarily chained to a toilet. Fortunately, there's a flicker of light at the end of this dismal tunnel: After delivery, no matter how bad it is now, the only nausea you will probably experience will be set off by a particularly stinky diaper.

Hyperemesis Gravidarum

Hyperemesis gravidarum (HG for short) is as grave as it sounds—involving excessive vomiting in pregnancy, as often as fifty times per day. Before that makes you lose your lunch, know that this nonstop vomit fest is rare, inflicting its own brand of torment on no more than 3 percent of expectant mothers. It is, however, one of the most common reasons pregnant women are admitted to the hospital.

HG can cause excessive weight loss, dehydration, injury to the esophagus, ruptured capillaries, and a host of other medical issues. More so than with regular pregnancy nausea, HG exacts a heavy financial, emotional, and physical toll on its sufferers during what should be a happy time—nearly 70 percent of HG sufferers miss work because of the illness. The psychological toll of HG is just as terrible, and not to be taken lightly. Unlike the many women who experience "normal" morning sickness in pregnancy, the lone HG sufferer is often miscast as being whiny or blowing the situation out of proportion, which couldn't be farther from the truth. (So even if this isn't happening to you, think twice before you write off your pregnant friend's or coworker's complaints.)

While morning sickness is merely unpleasant, hyperemesis gravidarum is beyond horrific for those who suffer its effects. Eating can trigger it. Smelling can trigger it. Blinking can trigger it. Breathing can trigger it. You are at the mercy of the porcelain gods—and they are not benevolent. It's important to consult with your doctor ASAP if you feel you're suffering from more than mere morning sickness. Should you be diagnosed with HG, the earlier the treatment begins, the better.

Unfortunately, nothing currently exists to stop HG from happening. See pages 124–5 for some suggestions that may, or may not, help. If you're diagnosed with this medical issue, your doctor will work

> Women who are carrying girls are more likely to suffer from hyperemesis gravidarum than those who are carrying boys.

with you to treat its effects and, hopefully, reduce its occurrences and symptoms. For milder cases, your physician is likely to recommend dietary changes, more rest, and antacids in the hope of settling that upchuck reflex that's been putting in some major overtime. For this reason, it's a good idea to keep a journal to track any specific foods or smells that might trigger your nausea.

> One Monday, a pregnant mom went to wake her mopey teenager for school. When she turned on the light, she noticed her daughter looked terrible and asked what was wrong. "I have morning sickness," the teen replied. The pregnant mom started crying and exclaimed, "How could you be pregnant?!" The surprised teen replied, "I'm not. I'm just sick of mornings."

For more severe cases, your doctor may recommend a short hospital stay. No need to worry: You'll likely receive IV fluids to counteract the dehydration that often accompanies frequent vomiting. In extremely severe cases, your doctor may recommend a nasogastric feeding tube, which enters through the nose and then ends in the stomach, delivering nutrients straight to where they need to go—no more pesky food odors or chewing necessary. Inconvenient and sucky? You bet. But given how you've been feeling, it may be just what you need to ride out the storm.

FYI ⇨ "What's that? My prenatal vitamin might be making my nausea and vomiting much worse?" 'Fraid so! If you suspect this might be the case, you may want to try liquid prenatal vitamins instead of traditional capsules or pills to see if the nausea subsides. Some women find that relying on whole foods for many of the vitamins and minerals found in the prenatal vitamins provides freedom from nausea. If you follow their lead, you can then supplement only those minerals and vitamins that are difficult to eat enough of on a daily basis (notably folic acid). Make sure your doctor is on board with these changes. She may even be able to prescribe a gentler nutritional supplement.

FYI ⟶ Morning Sickness or Something More?

If you're wondering if your newfound close connection to the toilet and trash can is normal or something you should be nervous about, consult the following descriptors to see where you stand (er, stoop).

NAUSEA & VOMITING IN PREGNANCY	VS.	HYPEREMESIS GRAVIDARUM
Occasional vomiting	vs.	Vomiting several times per day
No weight loss	vs.	Weight loss
You can eat some foods	vs.	You can hardly eat
Nausea and vomiting bothers you and makes you late for work	vs.	Nausea and vomiting devastates you and keeps you immobile for much of the day

See the sections on NVP (page 120) and HG (page 122) for more information on how to deal with either of these pregnancy side effects.

There is no one cure for NVP or HG—everyone is different and reacts differently to different foods and supplements. There are a couple of researched info bits, however, that may prove useful:

- **Think carefully before popping pills.** If your nausea and vomiting rates as only annoying, it may be safer to just deal with it instead of taking medication. Nearly 98 percent of prescriptions given to pregnant women for vomiting and nausea are not specifically labeled

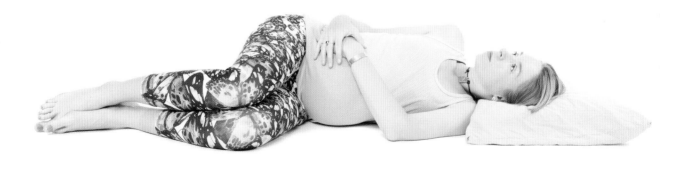

for use during pregnancy (unbelievable, right?). Consequently, class-action lawsuits are starting to crop up because of birth defects related to these morning-sickness prescriptions.

- **Rise and dine!** An empty stomach can cause waves of nausea. NVP sufferers should keep a snack on the bedside table and chow down before rolling out of bed in the A.M. to try to keep nausea at bay. Unfortunately, this advice doesn't work for HG sufferers, who can't help but have an empty stomach because they can't keep anything down!
- **Never take your prenatal on an empty stomach.** These potent vitamins commonly cause discomfort, because of either the iron content or the mere thought of having to choke down the super-size "horse pills." Consider switching to liquid prenatal vitamins to see if that helps.
- **Give your nose a vacation.** Odors are the most common triggers of nausea. Hyperolfaction, an incredibly intense sense of smell, is a symptom of NVP that causes even the most ordinary scents to be problematic during pregnancy (more on page 84). If you can avoid cooking, picking up after the dog, or breathing in perfumes, cigarette smoke, and other possible vomit-inducing aromas, you may be able to minimize your time spent hugging the can.
- **Time your meals wisely.** There are periods in the day when you feel better than others. Eat your largest meal and take your prenatal vitamins then.

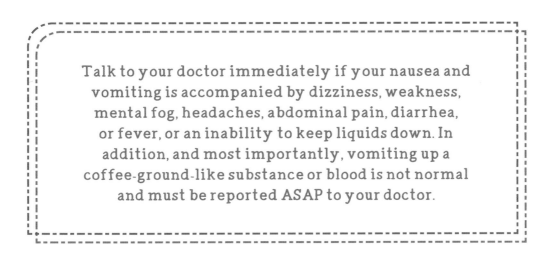

Talk to your doctor immediately if your nausea and vomiting is accompanied by dizziness, weakness, mental fog, headaches, abdominal pain, diarrhea, or fever, or an inability to keep liquids down. In addition, and most importantly, vomiting up a coffee-ground-like substance or blood is not normal and must be reported ASAP to your doctor.

Dehydration

Despite being filled to the rafters with more fluid than ever before, you can still get dehydrated if you aren't drinking enough water and other liquids. As discussed on page 122, vomiting can cause dehydration, which in turn causes feelings of nausea, creating a horrific, never-ending loop (like being stuck on a Ferris Wheel of Agony!).

Dehydration also causes constipation, fatigue, headaches, and a swarm of other unnecessary problems, including premature labor. The easiest way to check for dehydration is by the color of your urine: If it is darker than lemonade (say, the color of honey), that's usually a sign, but it can get tricky because of discoloration from prenatal vitamins. Your best bet is to simply keep track of your water intake and to drink as much water as possible (see page 127 for tips).

Many women find themselves limiting liquids because they dread being hitched to the bathroom (and being incontinent; see page 52 for more), especially during the night. Limiting liquids after dinner can help prevent that from happening so you can get a good night's sleep.

HOW TO ⇨ Drink More Water

Your bloodstream is the superhighway to your placenta, delivering nutrients and hormones to your growing baby. Since blood is mostly water, when you are dehydrated, your blood turns into sludge and the superhighway gets backed up in a traffic jam. How much water is enough? Most experts recommend about eighty ounces (or around ten cups) per day. Here are some hints to help you hit that goal:

- **Drink water all day**. Upon waking, top off a reusable bottle with water and sip on it during the morning. Refill it at noon and keep on sipping. Repeat until you've met your daily quota. If you become bored with plain old H_2O, try adding lemon, lime, orange wedges, fresh berries, or cucumber slices to your water for a refreshing twist.
- **Make other drinks count**. If you reckon water is only for fish, you can get your fill by drinking more palatable beverages, including decaffeinated coffee, herbal tea, unsweetened fruit juice, and milk.
- **Count foods, too**. Many foods contain lots of water—yes, watermelon, we're talking about you! But also honeydew, cantaloupe, and other types of melon as well as oranges, celery, bell peppers, tomatoes, lettuce, and cucumbers to name a few. Chow down.

Overachievers, take note: You can have too much of a good thing. Drinking too much water too quickly can overwhelm your kidneys and consequently dilute the electrolytes in your bloodstream, raising the risk of hyponatremia, a potentially life-threatening condition.

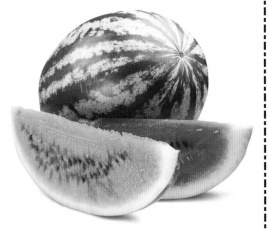

Anemia

Being iron deficient, or anemic, is all too common during pregnancy—it happens to nearly one in five women. Typical symptoms of anemia include weakness, dizziness, pale skin, irregular or rapid heartbeat, and trouble concentrating. In untreated cases, anemia is related to low birth weight and preterm delivery. It may also be a factor in some cases of postpartum depression experienced by new mothers. Anemia can usually be resolved or prevented with an iron supplement (prescription or over-the-counter) or prenatal vitamins, or by eating foods rich in folate, iron, and B12. Consult with your doctor.

Fainting, Lightheadedness & Dizzy Spells

Fainting spells were the pee sticks of the 1800s, back when an attack of "the vapors" was often the way that folks figured out a woman was "with child." We may have chalked all that fainting up to those cursed corsets, when in fact newly pregnant women can find themselves feeling faint or dizzy because of low blood pressure, low blood sugar, anemia, or dehydration, or even an increase in hormone production.

Feeling faint or dizzy can happen when lying down, standing up, or walking around (especially if it's hot outside), and in the shower or bath. Straining to cough, pee, or poop can sometimes be enough to make a pregnant woman get dizzy or faint. Drinking plenty of water and eating small, healthy meals and snacks throughout the day proves helpful, as does giving up on your skinny jeans—tight clothes (remember those corsets?) can cut off circulation and bring about lightheadedness.

Starting in the second trimester, you may find yourself prone to a more unexpected cause. Turns out lying on one's back becomes impossible for about 10 percent of pregnant women who find themselves dizzy, faint, or nauseous in this position. When you lie on your back, your heavily pregnant uterus puts pressure on the veins that carry blood throughout your system, creating circulation issues with potentially dangerous symptoms. In the most severe form, and if paired with any other unusual symptoms such as pain, vaginal bleeding, or heart palpitations, the effects are attributed to supine hypotensive syndrome. Should you experience such extreme symptoms, call your doctor immediately to rule out this larger problem.

Anytime you feel faint or dizzy while you are pregnant can be hazardous. Your main goal is to avoid a fall, so keep these points in mind:

- If lying down, turn to your side or try to sit up, which should alleviate much of the dizziness.
- If standing, sit down immediately and put your head between your knees (or put your chin in your boobs, depending upon how pregnant you are).
- Breathe deeply, and if possible, have someone open a window or turn on an oscillating fan or the air-conditioning, to improve air circulation.
- Have something to eat or drink in case the culprit is low blood sugar.
- If your clothing is tight, do what you can to loosen it.
- Wiggle your legs and toes to get the circulation going.
- When you get up from either a horizontal or sitting position, do so slowly.
- Don't ever be ashamed to call for help in getting up— this is one time in your life where it is totally OK to be the damsel in distress.

After years of infertility, Marie Antoinette, queen of France, was under tremendous pressure to produce a male heir. Shortly after childbirth, she fainted, and many historians believe that it happened because she was so shocked and disappointed to find out that she had delivered a girl.

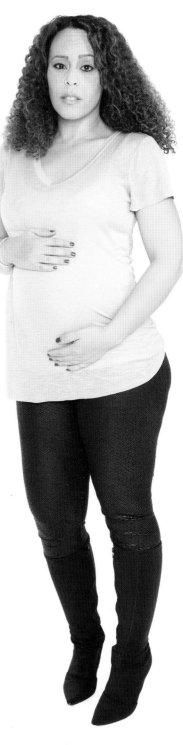

Eating For Two or Twenty-two?

The recommended caloric increase when you are pregnant is slight: only about three bananas a day worth of extra food. The theory that a pregnant woman is eating for two, and thus can eat as much as she wants because "it will all come off during breastfeeding," has been thoroughly debunked (sad, right?). Rather, it's not how much you eat but what you eat that counts. Studies show that the nutritional content—or lack thereof—of your diet can affect the health of your baby for the entirety of her life.

> Rapid weight gain—at the rate of over two pounds per week—can be a sign of preeclampsia. Check out page 4 for more information on this dangerous condition.

Sticking to just a few hundred extra calories a day may or may not be difficult for you, depending upon your relationship with food (and whether you are surrounded by superb cooks who derive joy from feeding a pregnant woman). Pregnant or not, food has emotional and social elements in addition to being a source of nutrition and sustenance. For some, ignoring the little voice in your head that's begging for a third helping of mac-and-cheese is easy, whereas for others (myself included), putting on the brakes is incredibly hard. Especially because we've been conditioned to think that pregnancy is essentially one long green light (as in Go For It)—and so you eat constantly, and with reckless abandon, to fatten up the baby.

Make sure to treat yourself to a little extra something, but within reason. And don't beat up on yourself if you go overboard every now and then. No pregnant person is perfect. This information is here because I wish someone had shared it with me. I was so excited to finally put on elastic pants that I ate everything anybody pushed in front of my face, firmly believing that I'd lose all the baby weight when nursing. Didn't happen! I was one of the few women I knew who *gained* weight while breastfeeding, mostly because I hadn't said no to any cravings for the ten months prior; thus telling my brain (and mouth) to stop eating everything in sight took quite a while. Mamma mea culpa!

Just do the best you can to treat your body like the temple it really is and not a fast-food dumpster.

▶ *While at the doctor's office, a pregnant woman asked, "I can't sleep at night without at least two cream-filled cookies. Is this craving normal?" The doctor responded, "Depends on what you are doing with them."*

Altered Tastes

One month you're a chocoholic. The next month you couldn't care less about the stuff. Pre-preggo, you may have sucked down so much diet soda that you imagined it running through your veins. Now when you take a sip, it's as though you're drinking liquid steel. Why have your best buds turned on you? Say thanks to your raging pregnancy hormones.

Turns out more than half of gestating women report changes in taste. Some pregnant women experience hypogeusia, which is when foods start losing their flavors completely. More common is dysgeusia, whereby foods you normally like suddenly taste metallic, salty, or even rotten. One-third of pregnant women find themselves dealing with dysgeusia in the first trimester, but the issue tends to dwindle in the second and third trimesters and disappear in the postpartum period.

Love sucking on lemons? You're not alone. But this acidic craving can cause a host of postpartum problems with your teeth. See if you can satisfy it with a glass of lemonade instead.

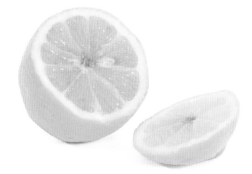

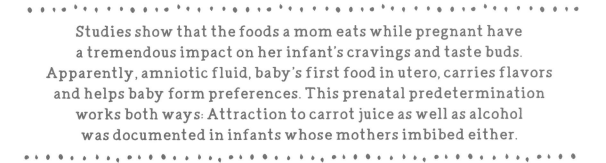

Studies show that the foods a mom eats while pregnant have a tremendous impact on her infant's cravings and taste buds. Apparently, amniotic fluid, baby's first food in utero, carries flavors and helps baby form preferences. This prenatal predetermination works both ways: Attraction to carrot juice as well as alcohol was documented in infants whose mothers imbibed either.

CRAZY CRAVINGS

Pass the chocolate-chip-cookie-and-pickle sandwich, please! When it comes to food cravings, 100 percent of women studied gave in to at least one insistent food desire during pregnancy, with sweets and fast food being the main culprits. While some cravings seem ridiculous, like olives and ice cream, others are more in line with general food preferences.

These cravings can shift throughout your pregnancy. Your taste buds may start out longing for the sourness of kimchi or lemon and end up craving the gooey sweetness of a fudgy brownie by the second trimester. Once you hit your third trimester, there might not be enough potato chips and popcorn in the world to satisfy your appetite for salt.

Quantity may be the wild card, as instead of one scoop of ice cream, the decadent preggo might find herself emptying out the tub in one sitting. Not surprisingly, a lack of willpower in the face of pregnancy cravings correlates with excess weight gain, but if you just can't put down the pizza and Oreos, you're in good company. Over half of pregnant women gain more weight than is recommended—including yours truly!

> What is a common pregnancy craving?
> For men to be the pregnant ones
> and not women.

Meat-craving Vegetarian!

Vegetarians often report craving meat in pregnancy, which is ironic considering many carnivores find they have an aversion to meat while pregnant. Many veggie preggos give in to their unfamiliar hankerings and start eating meat during pregnancy (even if they stop again after giving birth). But if doing so goes against your personal or religious beliefs, don't feel like you must make compromises because of the mistaken belief that your cravings are little red flags signaling your body needs meat (or whatever else). If you are concerned about your cravings, ask your doctor about checking for iron or other deficiencies.

Chalk Is *Not* a Snack!

Food cravings are normal, but pregnancy can make you do some pretty peculiar stuff—at least in the sense of sparking an intense desire to chew or suck on edible items with no nutritional value, such as ice, or even inedible items, including dirt, soap, chalk, clay, or paint. This condition is called pica and is often triggered by a nutrient or iron deficiency (see page 128).

Whatever you do, *do not* submit to any yearnings, no matter how intense, to eat things that are not food—even a tiny taste of laundry detergent or charcoal could pose a big problem for you and the baby. For instance, lead poisoning is common in pregnant women who eat soil because of an irresistible urge. And be careful with ice-crunching, as it can damage your already pregnancy-weakened teeth.

Pica is Latin for magpie, a bird known to eat many nonfood items.

If you're recovering from or still actively dealing with an eating disorder, let your doctor know and start seeing a therapist ASAP. Pregnancy brings tons of bodily changes that can trigger loads of emotions regarding eating, cravings, and the inevitable weight gain, so it's important to have support systems in place to help you deal—and without shame or guilt.

Heartburn & Indigestion

Pregnancy hormones prompt your stomach valve, the guardian that keeps acid out of your esophagus, to hit the snooze button. It doesn't help that your baby is crowding your stomach, which in turn pushes acid up toward your throat, irritating your digestive system and resulting in dyspepsia—the medical term for signs of indigestion such as burps and discomfort after eating. Another major player in this scenario is heartburn, that uncomfortable (or even painful) burning sensation in your throat. All of this is often accompanied by a little bit of regurgitation, meaning sometimes you're spewing tiny sparks of fire into your mouth. Good Times.

Here are some ways to head off heartburn:

- avoid bending over (gravity is not your friend when it comes to heartburn)
- keep your head elevated when lying down
- wear loose clothing so there isn't additional pressure on your stomach
- eat multiple, smaller meals instead of a few large ones
- don't eat late at night
- steer clear of juice, caffeine, fiery spices, and other heartburn triggers
- chew sugarless gum

Talk to your doctor about heartburn medications that are safe during pregnancy, notably antacids, which (as their name implies) counteract the level of acidity in your tummy and have been proven effective at reducing or eliminating pregnancy heartburn.

Unfortunately, heartburn is known to get worse before it gets better, with the third trimester being a nonstop acid trip for many (and not in a good way). Hang in there: It usually disappears immediately after birth.

Intolerances & Allergies

Does even the thought of drinking milk turn your stomach? Do grains get you gassy? Pregnancy can induce temporary food intolerances and allergies, most commonly for lactose, gluten, and eggs.

A food intolerance is a metabolic issue that may cause you to feel awful, but it won't land you in the ER. Your vigilance should align with the potential discomfort you'll experience, as intolerances by themselves do not affect the baby. That said, the side effects of indulging in food items that your body has become intolerant of, including diarrhea, aren't very healthy for either of you. Intolerances ebb and flow, so keep a stocked pantry and fridge to make sure you always have a variety of different, delicious foods to eat that won't give you grief.

A food allergy (like a peanut allergy), on the other hand, causes your body's immune system to kick in and can be life-threatening. Pregnancy may have triggered a new food allergy or a dormant allergy to flare up, so talk to your doctor ASAP if you suffer symptoms after eating or drinking that go beyond gas and stomach pain, to include: skin reactions such as tingling, swelling, or hives, or respiratory issues such as wheezing or difficulty breathing.

Allergies tend to get worse with repeated exposure. The moment you realize that food might be causing an allergic reaction, notify your doctor, who may prescribe emergency epinephrine to avoid anaphylactic shock in case of a serious allergic reaction, which could hurt the baby.

You will also need to learn to navigate various environments—work, restaurants, airplanes, among many more—to ensure that you're not exposed to the allergen(s). Your doctor might also refer you to a nutritionist who can help you plan meals and make sure yours is a well-balanced diet, especially if the list of foods to avoid exceeds the list of foods you know you can eat.

Food Aversions

It's almost guaranteed that, because of how hormones affect your taste buds and sense of smell, you are going to develop some food aversions while you are pregnant. In other words, the taste or smell of some foods (and sometimes the mere sight of food) will make you feel sick to your emerging stomach. Provided you're getting all the nutrients you and your baby need, let your aversions rule the day. For example, if the smell of eggs being cooked makes you heave, skip them for a few months to see if you feel better. But don't toss food that's not expired just because you don't want to eat it right now! Food aversions, like cravings, can evolve over the course of your pregnancy—you might detest the smell of ketchup this week and pine for it a month from now.

Peanuts & Pregnancy

Start spreading the news (and the peanut butter): The latest studies debunk previous reports showing a relationship between eating peanuts during pregnancy and your child developing a peanut allergy, asthma, or eczema. In fact, you may even be reducing her chance of developing nut allergies by exposing her to a possible trigger. Of course, if you yourself are allergic to peanuts, steer clear in pregnancy as you would at any other time and with any other allergy.

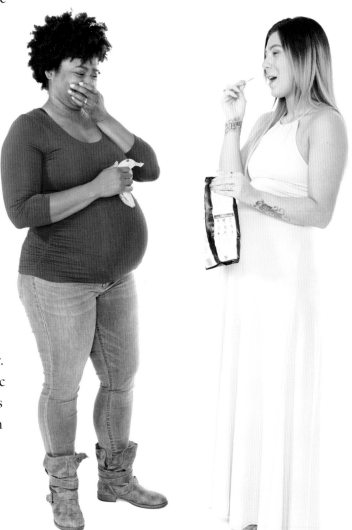

Gestational Diabetes (GD)

GD-it, you have GD! (Couldn't resist.) You're not on your own, either: Anywhere from 5 percent to nearly 20 percent of pregnant women have gestational diabetes. Sometimes it goes undiagnosed because symptoms are so like "regular" pregnancy symptoms. You may have unquenchable thirst, insatiable hunger, or fuzzy vision. You might pee a quadrillion times a day. You may also think these are just more baby-bump side effects, but your doctor knows better and tests you for gestational diabetes—and sure enough, your blood sugar is high, high, high.

Some moms-to-be have an increased likelihood of acquiring gestational diabetes (a matter for your doctor to determine), but no one is entirely safe. GD happens when your body becomes resistant to the insulin that your pancreas produces; specifically, your placenta is pumping out hormones that are interfering with insulin when it's trying to do its job, which is to keep your body humming along as it stores and uses sugar. When that extra sugar is allowed to float around in your bloodstream, it causes the high glucose readings that tell your doc you have GD.

Once you've been properly diagnosed, you'll quickly need a plan of action:

- **Your first priority is to not blame yourself.** It's not your fault! Stuff happens, and this stuff happened to land in your lap (or what's left of your lap).
- **Your second priority is to get your GD under control.** To do this, you'll probably have more frequent doctor visits, and perhaps even additional testing. It's entirely possible to get your blood sugar back on an even keel.
  - For mothers-to-be with a mild form of gestational diabetes, following a healthy meal plan and a doctor-approved exercise schedule, along with controlling your weight, may be enough to lower blood sugar levels.

- However, for some women, particularly those with a history of eating disorders, frequent dieting, and higher test results (as in the numbers suggest a more moderate to severe level of GD), the process can be much more involved.
- Your doctor will likely give you a treatment plan that may consist of nutrition education classes to create a sensible meal and exercise plan, and you'll probably be taught how to use a glucometer (a device for measuring your blood sugar) several times daily. You may also be prescribed medicine to get your blood sugar under control.
- **Your third priority is to refrain from "good" and "bad" labels.** That goes for the foods you eat, your blood sugar numbers, and yourself. A half-cup of ice cream and a slice of bread have about the same number of carbs; you get to choose. Your numbers provide information, but they don't reflect your value as a mom-to-be or as a human being.
- **Your fourth priority is to never skip a meal and to know the signs of low blood sugar.** If you're on medication or insulin, skipping or delaying a meal can result in low blood sugar (hypoglycemia); if you don't deal with it, you can die.
  - Symptoms of low blood sugar include shakiness, heart palpitations, anxiety, sweating/hot flashes, paleness, hunger, and confusion.
  - Educate your partner, friends, and coworkers about the symptoms and what to do if they crop up, because you might not be able to recognize low blood sugar when it's happening to you.

High blood sugar while you're pregnant is related to carrying a big baby. That can make delivery more difficult and put baby at risk for birth trauma such as shoulder dystocia. Sometimes, the baby can have low blood sugar at birth; while this condition usually resolves within the first one to three days of life, some newborns have persistent, and more severe, cases that require additional care.

Having gestational diabetes also means that you have a higher chance of developing type 2 diabetes later in your life, but you can cross that bridge if you come to it. To ensure that you are no longer diabetic after birth, be sure to schedule a follow-up glucose test about six weeks postpartum. Just remember: Sticking with the healthful habits you learn through your GD journey can help you avoid paying the steep toll of developing a more debilitating disease.

SLEEP

Pregnancy Fatigue

Within weeks of conception, most pregnant women find themselves feeling all washed up—the joke being that the lack of sleep and exhaustion during pregnancy is just preseason training for when you'll be tending to your newborn's nonstop needs. Right now, however, your fatigue is no laughing matter. Being extremely tired and yet not getting enough sleep can be a self-perpetuating cycle: Fatigue causes stress and lack of sleep, which leads to fatigue-related stress . . . and round and round it goes.

If it seems as if you're always worn out in the first trimester, believe me, there's a good explanation: Your body isn't building just a baby but also a whole new organ—your placenta. These tough internal workings leave your body with little energy to do anything else, so it's normal to just want to binge-watch Netflix. Making matters worse are complications such as low blood pressure and low blood sugar, both common during this time, as is nausea and vomiting—resulting in the inevitable pregnancy fatigue.

With any luck, you'll get a break from the physical causes of fatigue in your second trimester, when your hormones and placenta have settled into their new jobs. However, any spike in your get-up-and-go might be flatlined if you are under a lot of additional stress and strain (say, by working extra hours to bolster your savings account), which can sap your energy reserves.

By the third trimester, most women report that physical fatigue is again severe enough to disrupt their daily lives, and this is expected. Thanks to pregnancy and baby weight gain, by the final weeks you're essentially lugging around what amounts to a couple of sacks of potatoes, 24/7! Late-term fatigue also frequently stems from poor sleep quality due to physical discomfort or pain. Waking multiple times during the night because of heartburn, backache, having to pee, or baby's happy feet takes a toll on your daytime stamina, as do common third-trimester sleep disorders, all discussed in this section, so read on—and chill out!

HOW TO ⇨ Fight Fatigue

No matter what you do, or how hard you try, fatigue won't disappear entirely. That's just the nature of the baby-mama game. However, there are strategies to help you reclaim at least some of your lost energy:

- **Rest whenever you can.** Whether it's a ten-minute meditation at lunchtime or hitting the sack before sundown, you will want to take every opportunity to fight fatigue in ways you can control. Over half of pregnant women say they started taking daytime naps in the first trimester, so what are you waiting for?
- **Check for an underlying issue.** Anemia, hypothyroidism, and deficiencies in vitamin D or folic acid can all result in a high level of exhaustion, but a tired preggo generally can't tell the difference. Ask your doctor to test you for these or other reasons for extreme fatigue–and keep taking your prenatal vitamins.
- **Rule out sleep disorders.** Disrupted sleep makes for a disgruntled mama-to-be. Determining whether or not your daytime sleepiness is other than normal is hard to do on your own, so if it is causing you concern, mention it to your doctor. Sleep apnea, insomnia, and restless leg syndrome can each increase the risk for developing diabetes and also impact the health of your baby. See more on these sleep disorders on pages 147, 149, and 74, respectively.
- **Get moving.** Fact, not fiction: Exercise generally makes you feel less tired. Taking a brisk walk, swimming laps, or doing a gentle workout can deliver those feel-good endorphins that boost energy and promote a good night's sleep.
- **Delegate, darn it.** You don't need to do it all. Cut your chores and household responsibilities down to the bare minimum. Let your partner pick up the slack or just learn to live with a mess for a few months–it's better for baby and you than overexerting yourself to prove that you're Superwoman.
- **Eat little meals more often.** To combat low blood sugar, consume smaller, nutritionally balanced meals throughout the day to help keep your blood glucose level on an even keel and put more pep in your step.

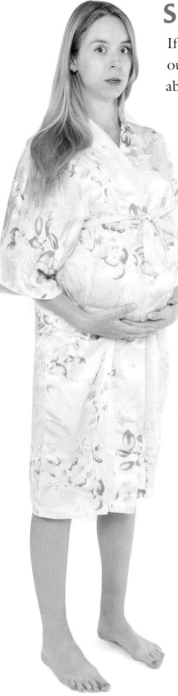

Sleep Paralysis

If you wake up and your mind tells you to open your eyes or get out of bed but your body is unable to move, you have not been abducted by aliens! You're just experiencing a discomfiting and often terrifying episode of sleep paralysis, which is not as uncommon as you might think (or hope). In fact, some studies find that sleep paralysis increases later in pregnancy. If you find yourself in a temporary stupor, wiggling just your fingers or toes instead of trying to move your entire body can help you snap out of it.

There is often no rhyme or reason as to why sleep paralysis happens in pregnancy, though some think it's prompted by a general rise in anxiety. Your mind and body are undergoing a lot of emotional and physical changes that can significantly impact your slumber pattern (keep reading this section for more on sleep, blissful sleep!). Luckily, sleep paralysis tends to disappear after you give birth—at least mine did!

> Be glad you're not dealing with sleep paralysis in the 17th century. Back then, sufferers were believed to be possessed by demons!

Sleep Orgasms

Having "the big O" while you catch some ZZZZs is one of the most incredible—and unexpected—of pregnancy perks. If you think teenagers have cornered the market on wet dreams, think again: More than one-third of women (pregnant or not) report having an orgasm while asleep at some point in their lives, and another 20 percent say they had more dreams of an erotic nature during pregnancy.

Sleep orgasms happen because, generally speaking, hormonal changes in the rapid eye movement (REM) phase of sleep prompt a pulsing sensation in your vagina, which in turn can spark unexpected orgasms. Think of these nocturnal shenanigans as hard-won rewards for enduring morning sickness, "cankles," and other pregnancy predicaments—and enjoy the ride!

Orgasmic births, while rare, are real. Instead of feeling waves of pain during labor, a few lucky women find that their contractions actually feel pleasurable, sometimes bringing them to the point of orgasm. Here's hoping that you are one of 'em!

Snoring

Even if you always slept soundly and silently before, don't be surprised if you start sawing logs like a lumberjack during pregnancy—an especially common happening in the third trimester. Gestational snoring (yep, that's an actual phrase) often happens because of swelling, or edema, which can narrow the openings in your upper respiratory tract (i.e., your nose and throat) and restrict the flow of air in and out. Because this swelling is akin to edema of the hands, legs, and feet (see page 2), chances are if you have any of those, your partner has probably already invested in a good set of earplugs.

Pregnancy rhinitis (or stuffy nose; see page 85), as well as extra tissue in your throat from weight gain (either before or during pregnancy), can also contribute to the narrowing of your upper respiratory tract.

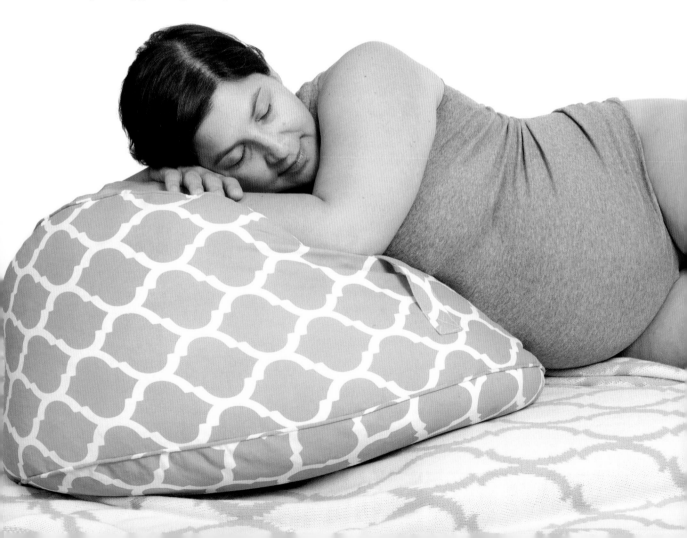

Snoring used to be considered just an endearing, albeit annoying, side effect of pregnancy. Now, recent studies have shown sleep-disordered breathing to be frequently paired with serious problems, including preeclampsia (page 4), gestational diabetes (page 137), and sleep apnea (an especially troubling problem discussed in the next section). If you stop breathing for several seconds, which can happen many times each hour when you have this disorder, both you and your baby are deprived of oxygen, possibly leading to low birth weight, delivery complications, and more.

You may well be asking: How on Earth will I know the difference between harmless snoring and harmful sleep apnea? It's tricky but not impossible to do, as discussed on page 147.

Avoid quickly bouncing out of bed like you did before you were pregnant—one wrong move can result in a dangerous fall. Upon waking, many pregnant women feel lightheaded, faint, or off balance, so take the time to sit up for a minute or two before carefully getting out of bed, preferably while holding on to something (or someone) for balance in case you're feeling woozy.

HOW TO ⇨ Snore Less

There's no single surefire strategy to keep you from snoring, but some tactics exist and are worth a try:

- **Sleep on your side**. Your upper airway is more likely to be restricted when you're on your back.
- **Open the airways**. Use nasal strips or (with your doctor's OK) a neti pot. Running a humidifier in your bedroom while you sleep can also work wonders.
- **Elevate your head**. To increase the flow of air, prop up your head on a pillow so that it's higher than the rest of your body.
- **Stay hydrated**. Drinking plenty of fluids helps loosen up the mucus in your nose and helps prevent the roof of your mouth located in the back (a.k.a. your soft palate or velum) from getting too sticky. The downside, of course, is that you'll probably need to pee more, which will interrupt your sleep, but you can always front-load the water as much as possible in the daytime.
- **Rule out other issues**. See page 147 for sleep apnea detection, and talk to your doctor if you think you might be suffering from that or other sleep disorders.

Is It Sleep Apnea?

If you are sawing some serious logs these days, you may want to make sure there's nothing behind all that noise. Ask your partner to study your snoring patterns for a few nights—he or she will likely be awake anyway!—and to check for these easy-to-spot symptoms of sleep apnea (in addition to snoring):

- pauses in breathing (even momentary ones)
- gasping, snorting, or choking noises
- shortness of breath (which may cause you to wake up)
- restlessness

During the day, the signs of sleep apnea are trickier to isolate because they can resemble general pregnancy fatigue:

- headaches
- fogginess (a.k.a. "mommy brain")
- excessive sleepiness

If you think you have sleep apnea, don't hesitate to get it diagnosed and treated. The doctor will typically conduct a few simple tests and then, if warranted, prescribe a special mask that's hooked up to one of several different types of machines, most commonly a continuous positive airway pressure (CPAP) machine. The CPAP pushes air through your nose while you sleep, clearing the obstruction that's preventing you and your baby from getting the oxygen you both need. Although wearing the mask may make you feel like a cyborg, and getting used to it may take some time, you will feel like a new woman once you get better-quality sleep.

> *A pregnant woman comes to bed looking radiant in a beautiful, lacy nightgown. She kisses her partner and says sexily, "You're not going to get any sleep tonight, so prepare to be completely exhausted tomorrow." Her partner smiles and says enthusiastically, "Sounds good to me." But before they can go in for another kiss, the pregnant woman flips over on her side, turns off the light, and says, "Great, because the doctor said that I have sleep apnea, and my snoring is going to be out of control."*

Nightmares

Herein lies the conundrum: You need all the sleep that you can get, but often your sleep comes with disturbing dreams. Some research shows that 70 percent of pregnancy dreams are unpleasant, usually revolving around such disheartening themes as being an inadequate parent, feeling undesirable or unattractive, or having a demanding labor.

Late in pregnancy, many women report dreaming of being trapped in a small space, thought to be an expression of how the mother perceives her baby to feel. (Stop worrying! It's warm and cozy in the womb.) In women who have suffered previous pregnancy loss, up to 80 percent have nightmares about complications in their current pregnancy and their newborn's health. Not surprisingly, first-time mothers are especially prone to nightmares.

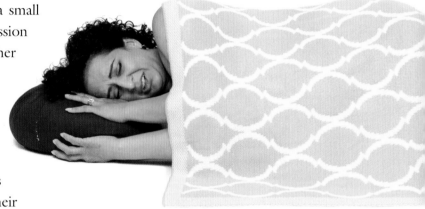

Resist the urge to take these "omens" literally. Your mind is fully prepared to play tricks on you right now, thanks to some fairly complex inner workings. Although you probably won't be able to stop nightmares from happening entirely, you can strive to reduce their frequency with physical exercise, doctor-approved massage, and meditation—all smart ways to promote a healthy pregnancy, too.

Although your pregnancy dreams are different from your nonpregnancy dreams, that doesn't mean there is anything wrong with you or your baby—so rest easy! Interestingly, at least one study found that women who had a greater number of nightmares experienced shorter labors and fewer complications when giving birth.

Insomnia

Some preggos have trouble staying asleep, but many more find it difficult to fall asleep in the first place—even when they are dead tired. Many underlying causes of insomnia, such as hormonal or metabolic changes, are admittedly beyond your control, but there are other possible sleep stealers that are not:

- **Your mood.** Anxiety, stress, depression, and other negative feelings and emotions can create a cycle of sleeplessness that only heightens these feelings. For your sake, and that of your baby, it's important to be conscious of fluctuations in your mood and emotional well-being. You can help regulate these changes through breathing techniques, exercise, and meditation. However, you may find that you need your doctor's help in addressing certain persistent symptoms. Either way, do not suffer in silence. Talk to your trusted confidants and ask for their support and guidance.

- **Hunger pangs.** If you usually eat dinner a few hours before going to bed, your baby might need a little nighttime "womb service." But don't trade those hunger pangs for heartburn pains brought on by eating too much food too close to bedtime. Instead, plan on a healthy after-dinner snack or small meal that will fuel your body until morning. Also, be sure to steer clear of anything caffeinated after lunchtime so you don't end up wide-eyed and bushy-tailed when it's time to drop off to sleep.

> Restless leg syndrome or leg cramps may be keeping you up at night, too. See page 74.

Your dreams will also never be sweeter than when pregnant. Thanks to your raging hormones, they're likely to be much more vivid and wacky than at any other time of your life. These intense visions just might be more memorable, too: Researchers have found that people recollect their dreams better when they wake up during the night, meaning all those trips to the bathroom for pregnancy pee could be improving your fantasy life.

- **Sleep habits.** Just because your hormones are out of whack doesn't mean your sleep schedule has to be similarly erratic. Strive for consistency: Going to bed at the same time each night will create a regular routine that promotes sleep. It's also better to avoid late-afternoon naps, or at least take them as early as possible—sleeping too close to your usual turn-in time can do more harm than good.
- **Your comfort.** Invest in whatever tools you need to help lull you into a deep sleep. Lots of pillows or a specialty wedge can prop you up, while a body (or lumbar) pillow can prevent you from rolling onto your back. Tucking a pillow or wedge between your knees can help relieve back pain; using nasal strips might clear your airways enough to drop into the snooze zone—and stay there.
- **Screen time.** Looking at your smartphone, tablet, computer, and other gadgets right before bed can prevent you from falling asleep and seriously disrupt your sleep pattern. Adjusting the brightness level to the dimmest setting will help in case you simply must check your e-mail or Instagram account before nodding off—but it's not as effective as resisting the temptation altogether.

If the above suggestions do nothing to help your insomnia, talk to your doctor about prescription and over-the-counter sleep aids that are safe to take during pregnancy.

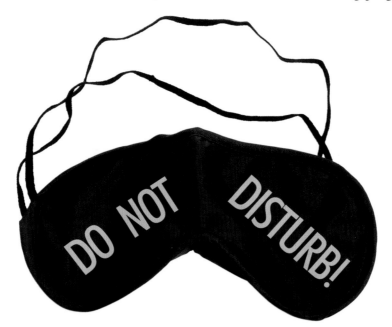

SEX & LOVE

>>> The evolution from showering each other in kisses as a childless couple to being showered in baby cries and baby crap is not easy on even the most solid of relationships. Not only do new issues spark during pregnancy, but problems that existed before baby can also heat up. But hey, at least the sex is smokin' (in the second trimester, that is)!

When Baby Makes Three: The Transition To Parenthood

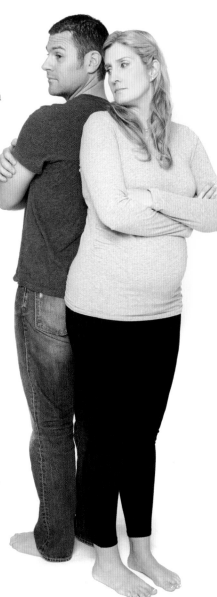

Partner problems usually start before the baby is even born. The shift in a relationship from couple to parents with the birth of the first baby is known as the transition to parenthood (TTP). This shift alters almost everything that makes up a romantic partnership, from your sex life to your bank account, and generally not in a good way.

Research shows that new parents tend to struggle to survive the first several years of child-rearing unless they put a lot of hard work into the relationship. That means improving the lines of communication, appreciating the value of give-and-take, establishing a mutual understanding of your needs and wants, and being a source of steadfast support for each other. In the long run, satisfaction levels among parental partners who put a premium on strengthening their relationships match up with those of couples who are nonparents.

If your relationship is in severe distress, you can (and perhaps should) seek avenues for outside support, including couples' therapy, which can often be a winning game changer.

Co-parent Education Is Crucial

Don't let your partner skip the parenting lessons! Plan to take at least one class or workshop together, even if you think you know everything already. Baby and childcare classes serve another important purpose besides being merely educational: They help you bond with your partner as co-parents from the very beginning on a level playing field, enriching you both (and your relationship) through equal informational opportunities and shared experiences. But the instructive value of these classes should not be overlooked, either. Not much attention is placed on nonpregnant partners, and studies show that they generally feel unprepared to be parents.

Parental partners who have a child between the ages of eight and twelve report the highest levels of satisfaction in their relationship. Some researchers call this the "golden age" of parenting. That's certainly something to strive for—and look forward to!

Studies also show that couples who attended parenting workshops together had greater relationship satisfaction than those who did not. If you can't afford or make time for actual classes, you can at least watch instructional videos at home, or maybe read this book together—anything to set the tone that parenting is a two-way street and a two-person job.

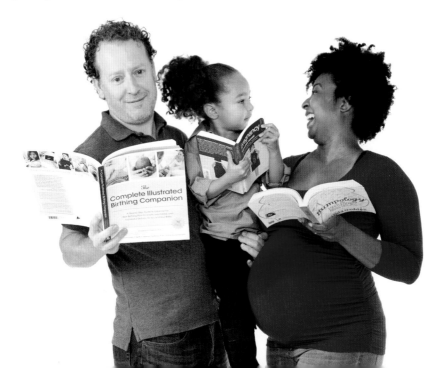

Depressed Dads-to-Be

Over 10 percent of dads become depressed during their partner's pregnancy, a number that is considered underreported due to stigma, shame, and a lack of awareness that father/partner prenatal depression even exists.

Your partner, like you, is more than likely feeling stressed, fearful, overwhelmed, and even confused by the shift in emotions, intimacy, and priorities, so encourage him to seek group or individual therapy, either alone or as a couple—or better yet both.

> The coin flips both ways: When moms have postpartum depression, between 25 and 50 percent of new dads also suffer from the baby blues, typically when the child is between three and six months old.

If you didn't catch on immediately to your partner's doldrums, give yourself a break. You're both going through so many changes that it's understandable not to notice. Now that you're aware of the potential for problems, consider whether your partner has

- a tendency to avoid work, family, or social situations;
- an inability to make decisions;
- physical issues such as headaches or stomachaches;
- drug or alcohol abuse;
- and/or moodiness, irritability, or flashes of anger.

It's essential that you and your partner be proactive about mental health on an individual basis and as a couple. Your partner's depression, and the strain it puts on your relationship, can take just as large a toll on your own emotional health as would suffering from your own bout of depression, which obviously wouldn't be healthy for you, your partner, or (most of all!) your baby.

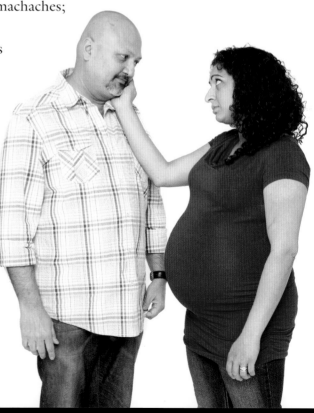

PregMANcy? It's Real!

You might not be the only one craving pickles and ice cream—leave some for your partner, too! Strange as it might sound, there have been instances where a man's body and mind mimic his partner's pregnancy developments.

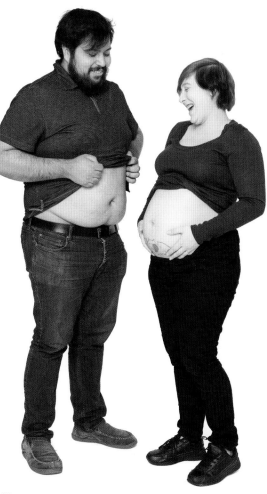

Couvade syndrome, the medical term for what is also known as a sympathetic pregnancy, is all too real—usually popping up in the first or third trimester and spontaneously disappearing once the baby is born (whew!). It's not rare, either, but many men are too ashamed to talk about it, so it's hard to know precisely how often this phenomenon occurs. Some studies suggest that as many as half of American dads-to-be have some symptoms of a sympathetic pregnancy. Emotional symptoms, such as mood swings, are the most commonly reported, but a good 20 percent of men have at least one physical symptom as well, ranging from insomnia and flatulence to back pain and morning sickness. There is even some evidence that men with couvade syndrome experience hormonal changes, right along with their pregnant partners. (That's a lot of hormones for one household!)

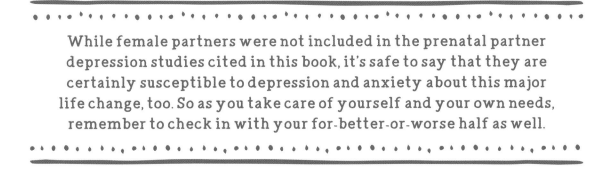

While female partners were not included in the prenatal partner depression studies cited in this book, it's safe to say that they are certainly susceptible to depression and anxiety about this major life change, too. So as you take care of yourself and your own needs, remember to check in with your for-better-or-worse half as well.

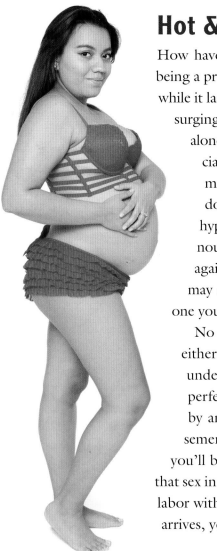

Hot & Horny Mama!

How have you gone from having a perfectly normal sex drive to being a preggo with the libido of an eighteen-year-old boy? Enjoy it while it lasts! In this case, at least, all that extra blood and hormones surging through your body are doing something that benefits you alone, rather than the baby. All your nerve endings—but especially those in your nether regions—are on high alert. What's more, the extra vaginal discharge ruining your underwear doubles as a sex lubricant. Your clitoris may be swollen and hypersensitive, just like your breasts, lips, and other erogenous zones. You want sex. You want it now. And then maybe again in an hour. If you don't typically orgasm during sex, you may start doing so now. Think of it as a delightful dividend—one you most definitely deserve.

No need to worry about knocking down baby's front door, either: Multiple studies have shown that so long as there are no underlying health issues (see next page), having intercourse is perfectly safe throughout pregnancy. Your baby is protected by amniotic fluid as well as a cervical mucus plug that keeps semen or lubrication from entering your uterus. And not that you'll be needing any extra incentive, but there's a slight chance that sex in the last week of pregnancy may even make for a smoother labor with less need to induce. Enjoy it while you can—once baby arrives, your sex drive may take a, hopefully temporary, nosedive.

Triplet brothers are in the womb discussing what they'd like to be when they grow up. One pipes up and says, "I want to be an electrician, so I can install some lights in here." The second boy replies, "I want to fix the pipes in here, so I want to be a plumber." The last one angrily yells, "I wanna be a boxer!" The other brothers ask, "Why's that?" He answers, "So I can beat up that crazy bald guy that always comes in here at night and spits on us."

When You Have To Say No To Sex: Doctor's Orders!

If you have a pregnancy complication such as spotting (page 59), an incompetent cervix, early dilation, or low-lying placenta (placenta previa), you may be cautioned against having an orgasm during sexual activity, and even from engaging in any form of anal and vaginal intercourse. Some doctors shy away from this discussion, so you may have to bring it up yourself. It's perfectly natural to ask for clarity about any medically proscribed limits on your sex life before writing all play off entirely (or before breaking out the *Fifty Shades of Grey* moves).

Over 60 percent of women report getting busy with their baby daddy in their third trimester.

Speaking of gray . . . sometimes there are gray areas where you may be allowed to have certain forms of sexual activity and even very gentle intercourse. But it's best to have this conversation with your doctor rather than figuring it out on your own. After all, you clearly had sex to get to where you are now, so the topic isn't exactly taboo (no immaculate conception here!).

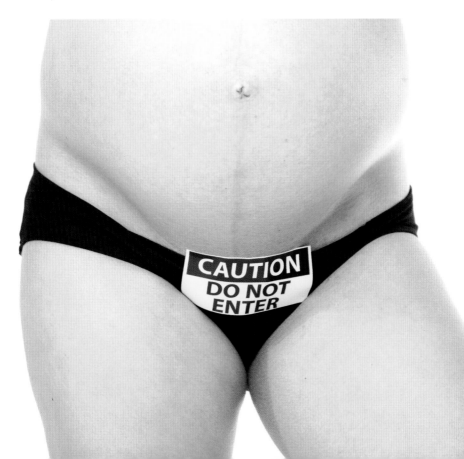

Best Pregnant Sex Positions

Every couple has their go-to positions. Over time, your sexual dance becomes perfectly choreographed. You anticipate each other's moves, you take turns leading, and your rhythms synchronize. At some point in your pregnancy, though, that effortless pas de deux disappears and you each feel like you have two left feet. Don't fret. With a bit of trial and error, you'll be tripping the light fantastic once again. Here are some tried-and-true positions to get you started. Some may already be part of your repertoire.

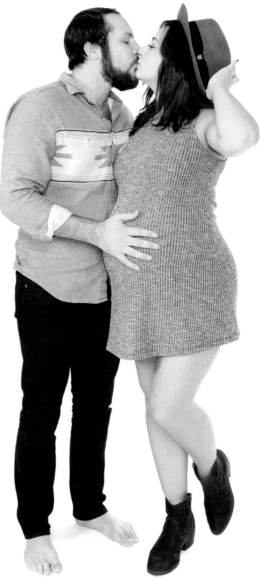

- **Spooning.** Lying on your side takes the pressure off your baby bump. With penetration from behind, you both have wiggle room to find the angle that sends you over the edge.
- **Doggy style.** When you're on your hands and knees (or elbows and knees), you're perfectly positioned for rear entry with your partner in a kneeling position.
- **Stirrup style.** Scoot down to the edge of the bed and raise your knees as though your feet are in stirrups (yep, just like at your many pregnancy checkups), with your partner standing at the ready. If you need to adjust your height, put pillows under your butt. For added traction and support, you can put each of your feet on a chair placed against the bed.
- **On top (a.k.a. cowgirl).** You know the drill— and you get to control the angle, speed, and depth for a change.
- **Reverse cowgirl.** In a spin (or about-face!) on the above, turn toward your partner's

feet, putting your hands on his thighs for stability. Bonus point: There's plenty of room for your belly.

- **Against the wall.** Standing with your hands (or elbows) against the wall and your feet spread, your nether region is completely accessible for penetration.

These are just some of the many positions to explore and adapt to conjure up your own favorites. Of course, oral sex and hand jobs are always options, too—whatever works for you when you're with child.

If you're feeling less-than-your-usual-sexy self because you've gained weight or developed a few new curves, you need to trade in your negative self-talk. Instead, form positive affirmations that allow you to celebrate the wonderful power of your body to create and nurture the life growing inside of you. There's nothing sexier than that.

Condom Common Sense

Just because you can't get pregnant while you're already pregnant doesn't mean you should put away the condoms, especially if you are not in a monogamous relationship. There's still the possibility of contracting sexually transmitted diseases (STDs) and infections (see page 56 for more on STDs), which only condom use can help prevent.

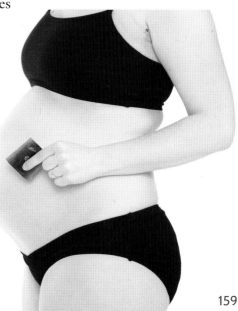

Pregnancy is a great time to encourage your partner to get tested for STDs so you can have absolute peace of mind—and he can show solidarity with the hundreds of needle pricks and blood tests you'll encounter during these next few months. And if something does turn up and it is treatable, you'll be able to cure the problem and keep from being infected (or reinfected).

Sex vs. Intimacy

Sex and intimacy are only kissing cousins, not identical twins. If you or your partner isn't interested in playing around, or you can't get busy because of doctor's orders, there are countless ways to feel incredibly close to each other—and to express your mutual love and attraction. Check out these ways to kindle your intimacy *sans* sex:

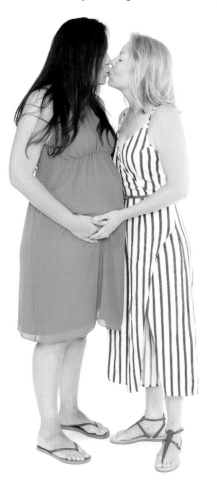

- **Nonsexual touching.** Ah, the beauty of foot massages by your one and only, holding hands at the movies, or—best of all—having an aromatherapy potion rubbed onto your baby belly. Pure bliss.
- **Love letters.** Tuck a note in your partner's lunch. Send a text listing three qualities you're grateful for. Tape your sonogram image to the bathroom mirror.
- **Day trips.** Spend an afternoon at the museum. Take a walk on the beach. Pack a picnic and head to the park.
- **Date nights.** Treasure baby-free time and take in a play. Go skinny-dipping at midnight. Win a stuffed animal at a carnival.
- **Simple pleasures.** Cook a gourmet meal together. Snuggle on the couch and stream a whole season of your favorite TV show. Take a class together that's not related to pregnancy and childbirth.

Don't be surprised if your partner notices a slight (or not-so-slight) difference in your flavor now that you're a mom-to-be. Reports have it that men find the taste of their pregnant partners more metallic or salty during oral sex than when the women were not pregnant. There's not much (if anything) you can do about this except to give your partner a heads-up before heading down there—and then forget about it!

When Your Partner's Not Into Sex With a Preggo

Talk about bad timing. Chances are your hormones have you feeling hornier than usual, but your partner puts you off and makes excuses for not being in the mood. You're understandably devastated. What should you do? First things first: Don't blame yourself. When partners avoid sex it says volumes about them and zero about the moms-to-be. So, what's up? Here are some possible explanations and work-through tips:

- **Your partner is turned off by your changing body.** This is proven to be the exception to the norm, because studies show that most men find their pregnant partners even more attractive, even if they don't want to have sex with them for the reasons below. (As yet, there are no comparable studies for same-sex couples.)

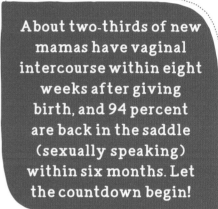

About two-thirds of new mamas have vaginal intercourse within eight weeks after giving birth, and 94 percent are back in the saddle (sexually speaking) within six months. Let the countdown begin!

- **Your partner is fearful of hurting the baby.** Your baby is well protected in the womb. Unless there are complications and your doctor advises against it (see page 157), sex poses no threat. Fight ignorance with facts. Invite your partner to read this section on pregnant sex, or have him/her join you in a discussion with your doctor about the ability to have a normal sex life.
- **Your partner is simply stressed out.** It seems like you're the one going through all the extreme transformations, but your partner might be experiencing anxiety, too, what with all the worries about money, parenting responsibilities, and other life-changing matters. Just strive to keep the lines of communication open and to discuss your anxieties so you can problem-solve together.

If you can't seem to bridge the sexual divide, seek out workable work-arounds. If penetration is the sticking point, there's always oral sex and mutual hand jobs. If your partner's just not feeling it, try a bit of foreplay; cuddling, hand-holding, and kissing can spark intimacy when you least expect it. Then there's always masturbation—break the ice by inviting your partner to watch (and vice versa).

Breaking Up During Pregnancy

Partners leave their baby mamas high and dry for a zillion different reasons: They're scared. They're immature. They're selfish. They're control freaks. They're all of the above. Then again, you might have to do the breaking up, especially if you're in an abusive relationship (see page 167). Whatever the reason, at the end of the day you've got to look to the future, not to the past. Becoming newly single during pregnancy has its challenges, but they're not impossible to overcome.

It's time to start making some lists, even if that's never been your thing. First, jot down everyone in your support network who can offer some type of help:

- family members near and far
- close friends and those you are in contact with via social media
- trustworthy coworkers and other confidants
- church members or other community folks
- meetup groups or other sources of support for single moms
- your doctors and other healthcare providers
- anyone else who comes to mind (think hard!)

Now is not the time to be prideful or to indulge your independent streak. You're going to ask for help. A lot of help. And people love to help a mom-to-be, especially one that has just left a horrible relationship.

Bad relationships are bad for baby. Children, including infants, have been shown to suffer long-term when raised in an environment lacking in warmth, cooperation, and effective co-parenting.

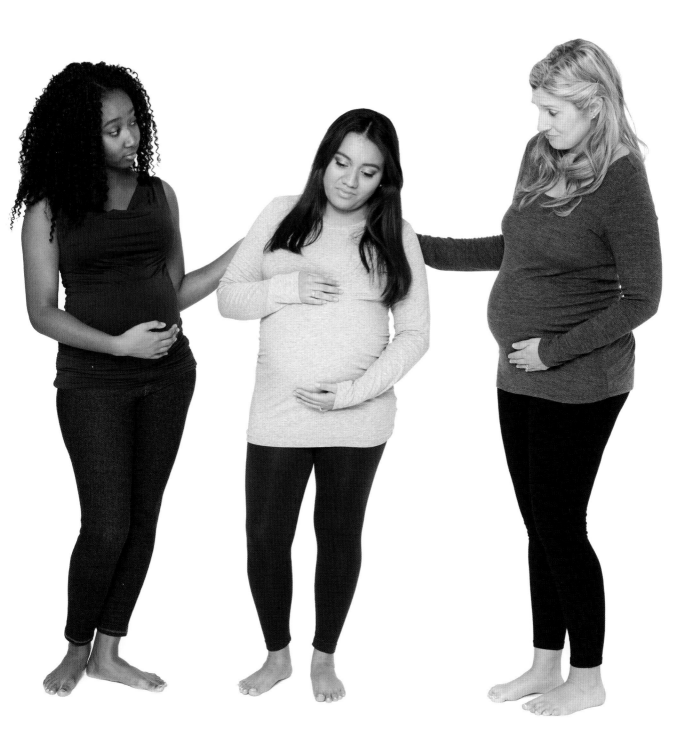

Next, take inventory of all the specific types of help you'll need through the remainder of your pregnancy, during labor and birth, and for the baby's first few weeks at home. Here's what you'll need help with while pregnant:

- doctor's appointments
- childbirth and parenting classes
- coming up with a birth plan
- decorating for the baby
- venting and expressing your feelings (good and bad)

Here's what you'll need help with during labor and delivery:

- childcare for your other children (if any)
- transportation to the birthing center (and a backup plan)
- creating a birthing environment that supports you
- a photographer/videographer for the big moment
- calling and texting everyone who should be contacted

And here's what you'll need once baby is born and you're back home:

- someone to spend the first several nights with you
- people who will deliver meals, run errands, do laundry, etc.
- childcare backup

If you're planning on being a solo parent, you've got loads of company: Nearly half of all pregnant women are intending to go it alone. Many of these women do maintain some sort of romantic relationship with the baby's co-parent, but they will still bear the brunt (or all) of the baby-rearing responsibilities themselves.

The first people you turn to might be your BFFs or your closest kin. If the stars align, you'll have core comrades who can implement your plan and make your life easier. If not, reach out far and wide. People will step forward and gladly ease your burden. You may also want to consult a few professionals along the way:

- If you're feeling paralyzed or overwhelmed, a professional therapist or group therapy can help you get moving again.
- The HR department at work can help you figure out how much paid sick-day and vacation time you have, the company's maternity leave (if any), when you're eligible for short-term disability, and how to apply for those benefits.
- An attorney can help you establish legal parenthood (and custodial parenthood for the baby's father), and start the ball rolling on getting child support.
- A doula is a professional birth partner who can take the place of your ex, or who can work alongside your chosen birth partner, in providing added support before, during, and after delivery.

You'll want to tap into the many resources that are available to help you and your baby thrive. The ones on pages 192–3 are all excellent places to start. And yes, thriving is absolutely achievable. After all, what do Olympian Michael Phelps, singer Barbra Streisand, musician Christina Aguilera, and presidents Barack Obama and Bill Clinton have in common? They were all raised by single mothers. Who knows to what heights both you and your own child can soar? The sky's the limit!

When It Just Doesn't Work Out: Child Support

Unlike in Hollywood, life isn't always punctuated with confetti and happy endings. If your baby partner is AWOL, the last thing you want or need to deal with after birth is endless paperwork. Find out if your state allows you to file in advance (while still pregnant) for child support, which is a mixture of court-ordered monthly payments and benefits such as health insurance the parent who does not live with the child must provide.

Even though the support won't begin until the baby is born, filing ahead helps to speed up the process. This is especially useful if there is hesitancy or outright denial by the baby's father, in which case you may need to establish paternity through a genetic paternity test. Beginning the process now rather than later might also wake him up to the fact that there really, truly is a baby on the way. So the earlier you get started, the sooner you can fall into a healthy, safe, and financially secure routine for you and your child. See page 192 for resources to help you with the filing process.

You may be hesitant to file for child support out of embarrassment, or if the baby's father asks you not to, but while the system is far from perfect, it is the best way to protect you and your child from relationship ups and downs that can directly affect your financial (and emotional) well-being.

In case you are hedging your bets, 30 percent of parenting couples who never marry break up within five years of having children.

166

Signs Of Abuse

Abuse can involve hitting, slapping, and much, much worse—or it can look a great deal different. Verbal, emotional, sexual, and financial abuse is just as destructive to your welfare as a punch to the stomach. If your partner humiliates you, calls you names, threatens you, or keeps you from your support system, that's abuse. If you aren't allowed access to your money or credit, that counts, too. And if your partner forces you to have sex that you don't want to have, he's crossed the line—and odds are he'll cross it again and again.

Your partner could be abusive if he/she is:

- jealous of any time you spend with your girlfriends or coworkers
- preventing you from seeing your family or friends
- calling you names or otherwise making you feel worthless
- controlling your money
- threatening to hurt him/herself if you leave
- punishing you by hitting or hurting you
- wrongly accusing you of cheating
- threatening you or the people you love
- keeping you from going to work
- sweet to you one minute and mean the next
- trying to convince you that you could not survive without him or her
- forcing you to do things (anything!) that you do not want to do

Pay attention now, because here's the bottom line: Listen to your gut. If you don't feel safe with your partner, you're not safe. You should never feel afraid of, or bullied by, your partner. You need to tell someone, you need an exit strategy if you're in danger, and you need to find a place to stay—and there are many safe havens for women just like you. Turn to page 192 for help finding these resources you need.

If you need help dealing with an abusive relationship, call the National Domestic Violence Hotline at 1-800-799-SAFE for 24/7 confidential support.

Abuse Is Not OK—Get Out!

No one has the right to hurt your body or your mental and emotional health. Although your doctor might not ask you about abuse, that doesn't mean it isn't an important issue. Abuse and violence are, unfortunately, extremely common during this vulnerable time: One in four women report emotional abuse from their partners while pregnant, 13 percent are physically abused, and nearly one in ten suffer from sexual abuse. In addition, over 30 percent of abused women are assaulted by their partners for the first time during pregnancy. Unfortunately, the number of pregnant women who suffer from abuse is probably much higher. Some (many?) women are often hesitant to report abuse either because they don't see themselves as victims or because they blame themselves for the abuse.

Hear this: There is no such thing as a typical victim of abuse—it can strike pregnant women of all religions, races, nationalities, ages, sexual orientations, and socioeconomic and educational backgrounds. There is also no one type of abuser. The emotions and life changes that pregnancy brings about, especially when your partner does not feel prepared for or is not especially excited about having a baby, often boil over into verbal, emotional, sexual, and physical abuse (see page 167 for more on the different types of abuse).

Abuse usually follows a predictable pattern: Tension in the relationship builds up over time, the partner becomes violent toward the pregnant woman, and what follows is a period of calm in which the violent partner tries to get the pregnant woman to make up with him by being gentle and loving and apologetic. Then the cycle begins all over again.

Whether it is the first or the fiftieth time that you've been abused, you and your baby deserve protection—as scary as it might seem to speak out about it, and as much as you may think you need your partner to be involved in your child's life. Many women find that being pregnant gives them the strength to leave their abuser, and with good reason—to keep their babies out of harm's way.

The sooner you make your move, the better off you will be—things will not get better once the baby arrives, no matter how many promises your abusive partner makes. In fact, partner violence tends to increase right after childbirth, and there is also a strong link between partner abuse during pregnancy and eventual abuse of the child(ren). Turn to page 192 for resources to help you safely leave your abusive situation and find the support you need.

> Fifteen percent of women with unwanted pregnancies suffer from partner abuse, compared to 5 percent of women who intended to get pregnant.

If you became pregnant against your will, either because your partner wouldn't let you use birth control or used emotional or physical tactics, you are a victim of what is called reproductive coercion, a form of domestic violence that strikes nearly one in ten women. Because reproductive coercion is usually not the only form of abuse in the relationship, getting out before the situation escalates is your best recourse. Act now and be safe.

TRUE STORY:
I LEFT MY ABUSIVE HUSBAND WHILE PREGNANT

BY ANONYMOUS

Fourteen weeks into a planned pregnancy, my well-known, Ivy League-educated, charming attorney husband tried to strangle me to death. He had a prior history of abuse with other women that he glossed over, and I didn't take seriously. Big red flag. He'd been arrested a couple of times for domestic violence, but he made it sound like his ex was exaggerating the abuse as a custody weapon. I knew he had a temper, but we had been together over two years and he had always controlled it. When I became pregnant, however, things changed. That's when the verbal abuse began to escalate until that fateful Thursday night. We'd argued before, and he'd been moody, but he'd never hit me before.

He told me that his physical attack was my fault. I had said something teasing, and he decided I had to die. Luckily, he didn't kill me. I had taken some Krav Maga classes long before and I remembered how to break a hold like that. I was able to get away and I immediately drove to an emergency room because I was having trouble breathing. At first, I was reluctant to talk about it, but they called the police. I hear so many stories about how the police are unsupportive or blame the victim, but in my case, they were really nice. No blaming me. I don't think they even asked if we'd gotten into a fight. The police called in the domestic violence advocates, and they let me stay at their secret shelter and went with me to the judge to obtain an order to protect me from further abuse. Friday afternoon, less than twenty-four hours after he had tried to kill me, the police forcibly removed my husband from our house. He was in his pajamas, eating ice cream on the sofa, watching Oprah. The police told him to never come back, and they continued to check up on me over the next few months.

I never saw him again. The story of Laci Peterson, the pregnant woman murdered by her husband in 2002, loomed large at the time, and I felt very afraid for a long time and was terrified that he would come back. I told everyone with ears what he did. I did not keep it a secret. That's one piece of advice I have for anyone in this dreadful situation–don't hide the truth. I really made it impossible for any kind of reconciliation to happen.

I didn't know at the time how much domestic violence increases when women are pregnant. It's frightening. Women are vulnerable when pregnant, more so than when we are not. Because I had quit my job to focus on getting pregnant, I was struggling to make ends meet. What's more, he had cleared out my checking account, leaving me just $320 total. It was rough. Not having a viable financial plan was messy and difficult.

That said? If you are in a similar situation, your life is at stake, so you need to be safe. A lot of people stepped up to help (that's another piece of advice–ask for help). I am lucky and not lucky. He never came back, and I never looked for him. I never asked for child support. It's never easy financially or emotionally, but I have to believe that my current situation is better off than my son growing up with him as a father. My son is now ten years old. He looks just like his father, but that's where the resemblance ends.

MENTAL HEALTH & STRESS

You might have peed on a stick a few months after a one-night stand, praying it was just a stomach bug, or you may have spent years planning and saving for this baby. Whichever way you've ended up pregnant, the combination of physical, emotional, relationship, and financial strains that comes with impending parenthood can cause deep-seated anxieties to fester, fear to percolate, and stress levels to overflow. You will both laugh and cry over the next few months, often at the same time and for no reason at all. Read on to explore what might be going on and what you can do about it—and know that you are not alone.

Blessed To Be Stressed

A healthy third-trimester woman has the same levels of stress hormones as a nonpregnant person suffering from major depression. But that's not actually a bad thing! Studies show that, oddly, those hormones seem to benefit the fetus and may even be preparing your mind for motherhood, so all the worry must be worth it!

Pregnancy Brain

Is pregnancy making you feel like you can't remember anything, even the sentence you read just seconds ago? Is pregnancy making you feel like you can't remember anything, even the sentence you read just seconds ago? (Ha, gotcha.) Tricks aside, pregnesia (a slang term for pregnancy amnesia) is valid: Studies show a legitimate decrease in short-term memory and cognitive function in pregnant women.

> *A pregnant woman asks a new mom, "Does pregnancy affect a woman's brain?" The mom replies, "I don't remember."*

Perhaps you've stared confusedly at your partner for a few seconds before snapping out of it and remembering who he is. Or maybe you've lost your keys for the tenth time this week. You're apparently just one of the crowd: Brain fog and forgetfulness affect most expectant women. Fascinatingly, your brain is literally getting smaller as your belly enlarges, with significant shrinkage starting as soon as your placenta attaches and continuing until birth. The memory center of the brain, or the hippocampus, is being downsized, and pregnesia increases with each trimester.

There is some good news, though: Unlike your body, your brain will quickly rebound after delivery without any intervention on your part. And while pregnancy brain may be a bummer, you can be stoked knowing that your mommy mind will be better than ever. After giving birth, research shows women develop mentalities that are bolder, more empathetic, and more emotionally resilient—all part and parcel of being a Supermom.

Fatigue vs. Pregnesia

A changing brain is not the only reason your thinking is muddled in pregnancy. Sleep deprivation and poor sleep quality can lead to a lack of energy, brain fog, and absent-mindedness. Check out the sleep section starting on page 139 for ways to combat fatigue.

Fatigue and depression can have similar symptoms in pregnancy, making it hard to tell which is which. Any issues that might make someone depressed, such as being out of work or lacking an emotional-support network, have been reported as causing pregnant women to feel more tired during pregnancy. See page 178 for more on prenatal depression.

The New PMS: Pregnancy Mood Swings!

Moody, broody mamas-to-be can take cranky comfort in the fact that the unpredictability of their emotional state is not only normal, but entirely justified. Your monthly spell of premenstrual syndrome was preparing your body for a potential pregnancy until the fertilization dreams of your uterus were dashed, causing it to release the blood floods as a surrender flag and your hormones to retreat for another few weeks. Your new PMS, a.k.a. pregnancy mood swings, can follow a preggo all the way through the postpartum months, but tends to peak in the first trimester.

Debbie-downer feelings like being sad, tearful, irritated, snappy, or angry are the most commonly reported. However, pregnancy moods can also swing high with unexpected bouts of happiness. I got giddy around my third month, finding myself inadvertently laughing at almost anything that anyone said—and I could not control it. I would even get the giggles during live-broadcast interviews on serious topics. My giddiness was so extreme that one of my coworkers suggested I spill the beans about my pregnancy to my boss so I wouldn't get fired for not taking my job seriously! Thank goodness I did!

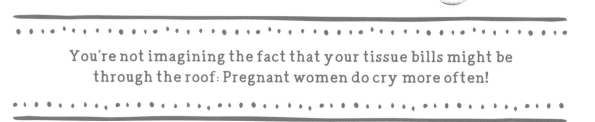

You're not imagining the fact that your tissue bills might be through the roof: Pregnant women do cry more often!

Beyond Hormones

While much of your emotional back-and-forth is due to pregnancy hormones, there are other factors at play as well. You aren't sleeping well (page 140), you've probably got heartburn (page 134) and back pain (page 70), and your brain often isn't working at full capacity (page 172). Adding insult to injury, you are probably worrying about something, or everything, and perhaps rightfully so. Here are some of the more common nagging thoughts running through the minds of many pregnant women, all of which encourage mood-swing-causing stress, tension, panic, and a sense of isolation:

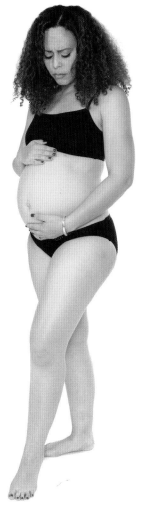

- My body is getting ruined.
- There isn't enough money.
- I'm not prepared to be a good parent.
- This is all just too much and I can't handle it.
- My partner might not love me as much anymore.
- I don't love my partner anymore.
- My baby might not be healthy.
- How is this baby going to get out of me?
- I don't know if I really want to be a parent.
- I don't want to repeat the awful parenting that I had growing up.

You may be ashamed of having these "terrible" feelings instead of being filled to the brim with nothing but joy and sunshine (and baby). But you are not alone in your thoughts during this stressful life event, and your tears are completely natural and normal, whether they are of joy or sadness or some strange combination.

What's more, you're not being the least bit selfish by putting yourself and your emotions first. Ignoring these feelings doesn't help, either; instead, try seeking counseling, either from professional therapists or psychologists, local support groups for mothers, or spiritual leaders. Or simply reach out to your partner and/or friends and family. See pages 192–3 for a list of resources to help you cope in a way that is best for you and your growing family.

The *H* Word: Hormones

The most frequently used word in this book is *hormones*. You may be tired of seeing everything explained as a side effect of hormonal changes, but it's really that simple (and complex!).

Think of your body as an airplane and your hormones as inevitable and unpredictable weather conditions. Your body's hormonal state is generally in smooth-sailing mode, but as soon as the egg is fertilized, alongside the baby a brand-new organ begins to develop called the placenta, which secretes a brand-new group of hormones, drastically changing your body's atmosphere from a gentle breeze with the occasional PMS thunderstorm to a constant ten-month-long torrential hormone hailstorm. Hormones often turn pregnancy into such a turbulent physical and emotional trip that you find yourself gripping your toilet seat with motion sickness as you hang on for dear life until making it to the hopefully successful crash-landing of birth. Whew!

That's one way of looking at your hormones. But another, more optimistic way is to accept them as your airplane-body's flight crew, with Human Chorionic Gonadotropin (HCG) as the captain of the cabin. Once your body officially books your passage to Babyland, HCG is the first hormone to greet you in pregnancy, and it's running the show.

The co-pilots, progesterone and estrogen, are extremely important, especially in the first leg of pregnancy, when they navigate your journey, dictating to your various body parts what they should and should not be doing. After the first trimester, progesterone and estrogen tend to take a back seat and let the rest of the crew of hormones run things, but they're always standing by in case corrective action is called for.

Rounding out Team Baby are oxytocin, prolactin, relaxin, testosterone, cortisol, adrenaline, and a cast of other minor characters that all play smaller, but important, roles in helping your body safely make it to Destination Mom.

Once baby is born, your hormones don't just shut off immediately. In the same way that a person feels jet lag for a few days after a long airplane flight, it usually takes a while for your body's hormones to calm down postpartum.

35-plus? You're Not Alone!

Elderly primigravida may read like a pasta dish with aged cheese, but it's in fact medical terminology for a first pregnancy where the mother will be thirty-five or older at the time of birth—and now there are more "elderly" mamas than ever before. Your doctor might use the slightly more appealing phrase "advanced maternal age," but at least it's not like it was in the 1970s, when older mothers were labeled "geriatric pregnancies" and considered to be somewhat freakish! Back then, the average first-time American mother was twenty-one years old. Today? She's twenty-six.

> At her annual checkup, a woman asked her doctor if she should have a child after thirty-five. The doctor responded, no, thirty-five children is enough.

Prenatal Depression

Do you feel like you might be dealing with more than just mood swings? Sometimes your emotions can be more complicated than garden-variety anxiety and a down-in-the-dumps slump. As mentioned elsewhere in this book (see pages 140 and 147), many indicators of depression are similar to general pregnancy symptoms, including fatigue, sleeping problems, and overeating. There are others, however, which are not so common. Ask yourself if you had any of the telling signs of depression during the past two weeks, including feeling:

- little joy in doing anything;
- hopelessness, sadness, or despair;
- bad about yourself, like you are a failure;
- unable to concentrate or focus;
- that you might be better off if you were dead;
- the urge to hurt or kill yourself.

If you answered yes to any of the above, does that problem(s) make it difficult for you to work, socialize, or take care of your home and family? If you answered yes again, know that you are not alone. Up to 20 percent of pregnant women are consumed by negative feelings for extended periods of time and suffer, often silently, with prenatal depression. It might seem easier to dismiss your depression as temporary or something to "push through," but if left untreated, prenatal depression can negatively impact your pregnancy, labor and delivery, and efforts at breastfeeding. It also increases the risk of postpartum depression.

Getting treatment is critical. Depression is a serious medical condition that requires professional help to conquer.

You don't have to be dysfunctional to be suffering from prenatal depression. In fact, many women present no signs to the outside world.

> Women who have suffered from depression or anxiety before becoming pregnant are at an especially high risk for prenatal and postpartum depression, but this risk is lowered with professional treatment. Surround yourself with a supportive team of doctors, family, friends, and other dependable souls to help you and your baby stay as healthy as possible.

If you are reading this book, you obviously want to take care of yourself, and you deserve to feel as healthy and happy as possible. Don't be embarrassed to talk to your doctor about your concerns so she can determine if it's just the baby blues or something bigger that requires treatment and monitoring.

Also, and importantly, don't think for one moment that you are "crazy," or that you did anything to bring this about. You can't figure this one out on your own, either; you're going to need help. Fortunately, assistance is widely available. See pages 192–3 for resources to get started on the road to feeling better as soon as possible. By working through these issues now, you could be preventing a more serious problem down the road.

If you are struggling with thoughts of suicide or self-harm in any way, put this book down ASAP and call the National Suicide Prevention Lifeline at 1-800-273-8255 for confidential and free support, 24/7. You can also turn to pages 192-3 for additional helpful resources to get you through this difficult time.

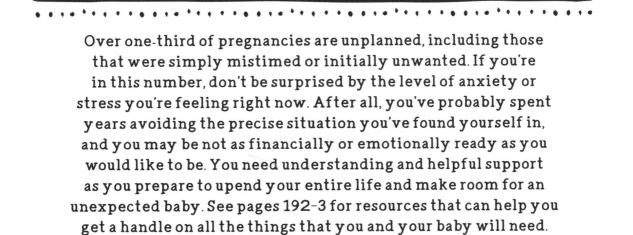

Over one-third of pregnancies are unplanned, including those that were simply mistimed or initially unwanted. If you're in this number, don't be surprised by the level of anxiety or stress you're feeling right now. After all, you've probably spent years avoiding the precise situation you've found yourself in, and you may be not as financially or emotionally ready as you would like to be. You need understanding and helpful support as you prepare to upend your entire life and make room for an unexpected baby. See pages 192-3 for resources that can help you get a handle on all the things that you and your baby will need.

Gender Disappointment

Many moms-to-be are fibbing when they say that all they want is "a healthy baby." In fact, over the past seventy years, thousands of women who were surveyed overwhelmingly desired a male if they could have only one child. On the flip side, female babies were requested by up to 80 percent of women who chose the gender of their fetus through sex-selection techniques—frequently to "balance out" their family if they already had one or more boys.

When trying to conceive my first child, I myself kept a wooden spoon and an infant dress underneath the bed in the hopes of convincing the fertility gods to send me a daughter, and the sight of my son's penis on the twenty-week ultrasound sent me into gut-wrenching, guilty sobs. Fortunately, I had a supportive partner and a strong base of brilliant women with whom I could be honest about my feelings.

Recognize that it is perfectly OK to be disappointed. It doesn't mean you don't love your baby, and it doesn't mean that karma is going to bring harm on your home because of your perceived pettiness. It just means that you are human and, like so many other aspects of pregnancy (and life!), your emotions are maddeningly out of control. Your feelings aren't right or wrong.

Discuss your thoughts and feelings with your partner, if possible, or acknowledge how you feel with an understanding family member or friend (or a therapist). Ask yourself why you are having these feelings. Are you disappointed because you grew up in a family with only brothers and are picturing yourself as a reluctant football mom? Did you imagine yourself choosing adorable outfits for a little girl? Bear in mind that even if you had gotten the sex of the baby you were hoping for, the child might not grow up with the stereotypical personality traits or interests of his or her gender.

Have faith in your ability to love any child you carry. Any guilt or discontentment you are feeling now will not last long. Once you give birth, you'll have a wonderful baby with his or her own quirky traits and a unique personality that will shine through in the years to come— and any gender disappointment will be a distant memory. If your disappointment does linger, however, help is available for you to get through that, too.

Instead of finding out whether your baby is "pink" or "blue," a growing number of women are on Team Green and choosing to wait until birth to learn their child's gender. This way, the thinking goes, they are minimizing the risk of any gender disappointment and putting the focus entirely on the excitement of the new family member, whoever she or he may be.

Bed Rest & Your Brain

Nearly one in five women will be put on "bed rest" during pregnancy. Sometimes doctors use the phrase as a catchall term for any kind of restriction on activity (like sitting more often or putting your feet up whenever possible), but more often it means what it sounds like—being confined to your bed for a certain amount of time, generally after twenty weeks.

Know this: Research has found that strict limitations on a pregnant woman's mobility are often not helpful in preventing problems or ending complications that affect the baby or the mother. Bed rest can also have a negative effect on the well-being of the mother, especially emotionally, opening the door to depression due to isolation, boredom, worries about the baby, feelings of being a burden on her household, and a general lack of freedom.

If bed rest is prescribed, be sure to ask your doctor if there are alternatives for your specific situation, or if the restriction can be limited. While on bed rest, it's a good idea to connect with online support groups (see page 193) so you can avoid any of the mental health issues that may stem from your confinement and that can inadvertently lead to birth and postpartum problems.

PTSD & Pregnancy

About 8 percent of pregnant women are also bravely managing post-traumatic stress disorder (PTSD), which comes on after a life-altering event and causes sufferers to constantly relive that event through flashbacks, nightmares, and unwanted thoughts that can pop up at random times. Most events are unrelated to pregnancy and include highly stressful and traumatic situations such as abuse, rape, assault, domestic violence, or being in a man-made or natural disaster. In one study, however, 40 percent of women who had a miscarriage were diagnosed with PTSD three months after the loss. Childbirth is also known to be a trigger in some women for a specific type of PTSD called postpartum post-traumatic stress disorder.

For many women, PTSD symptoms improve during pregnancy. Sufferers who experience new trauma during pregnancy, or those who are especially anxious about the upcoming birth, are more vulnerable to having PTSD-related complications throughout the pregnancy and into the postpartum period. If you have PTSD, it is very important that you seek professional help during pregnancy to minimize any chance of harm to yourself and your baby. Stress or risky behaviors common in PTSD sufferers include self-medicating with alcohol, cigarettes, or drugs.

> Most importantly, if you have any thoughts of hurting or killing yourself, your baby, or another person, you must seek help immediately!

Studies show that women with a strong support network are better equipped to handle PTSD during pregnancy and more likely to avoid postpartum depression, so now is the time to grow your social circle—along with the growing baby in your belly. You should also talk to your doctor ASAP and get the help you need.

Overcoming Childhood Abuse

If you were a victim of childhood abuse, especially sexual abuse, you are extremely vulnerable to PTSD as well as prenatal and postpartum depression. Some women question their ability to parent properly because of a lack of appropriate role models in their own families.

Remember: You *can* overcome your past. The fact that you are worried about this means that you know that you and your growing family deserve better. Stay strong. Put forth tremendous effort to educate yourself by attending parenting groups, asking professionals for advice, and seeking the counseling and guidance you need. These are just some of the ways to limit the influence of a painful background on your own family's future.

> Up to 90 percent of women turn to the Internet to find coping strategies to deal with depression. See pages 192–3 for resources that are safe and reliable.

OCD & Worrying About Harming Your Baby

All pregnant women worry about harm coming to their unborn baby, but excessive worry to the point of distraction can be a sign of something more serious: obsessive-compulsive disorder (OCD). Pregnant and postpartum women are more likely to experience OCD than others. If OCD is left untreated, it can have serious consequences for the baby and your ability to parent.

Pregnant women with OCD tend to be compulsive about the cleanliness of themselves and their environments, and to be preoccupied by fears of their babies being harmed in ways that are often unusual and extremely unlikely. Often, the most damaging aspect of OCD is the mistaken assumption that having these frequent, disturbing thoughts makes you more likely to harm your baby, and the fear that your baby will be taken away if you express those thoughts. Don't suffer in silence!

Get this straight: Thinking about horrible actions is not the same as acting horribly. Seeking professional help and being honest about what's happening is the best thing that you can do, both for yourself and your baby. Your doctor can help you manage your OCD and/or any other mental health issues—but first you must ask.

Coping With Loss

While most pregnancies result in healthy babies—and goodness knows I hope yours does, too—a sad-but-true fact of life is that many women, including myself, suffer a loss in pregnancy at some point in their childbearing years. Most losses occur before the twentieth week and are termed miscarriage; stillbirth numbers are much rarer, but are another sobering possibility.

It's important to discuss this heartbreaking reality because there seems to be a common belief among women that only a small percentage of pregnancies end in loss, so when it happens to them, or someone they know, it feels incredibly unfair—and much more so than it would if they only knew that the number is in fact closer to 20 percent.

Naturally, any loss is devastating to the individuals involved, but especially so when such loss is considered rare and therefore ends up being associated with feelings of guilt and shame. Here's another reality check: Most pregnancy losses stem from chromosomal abnormalities in the fetus and have nothing to do with the mom's ability to birth a healthy child.

This section is meant not to alarm you but to mentally prepare you to seek help in the event of a worst-case scenario. Nearly half of the women who suffer a loss during pregnancy experience PTSD (page 183). Others may suffer from depression, partner problems, and fears about trying to conceive again. These issues, and any others you might face after pregnancy loss, are difficult to overcome on your own. See pages 192–3 for resources to help you work through your grief, and if desired, continue along the path toward growing your family.

A recent survey revealed that because of the deafening silence that surrounds the topic of miscarriage, most women who have suffered a loss mistakenly believe that it is extremely rare. Not only will talking about your experience with others help you to process and heal, but it will also help to eradicate social shame and anxiety around a very common and natural, if devastating, part of procreation. When I opened up about my painful loss, "It happened to me, too" was the most common response I received from other mothers.

Rainbow Babies

Do not despair! Most women who miscarry are able to, over time, start or complete their family with a healthy pregnancy and birth. The odds are absolutely in your favor: Only about 5 percent of women have two miscarriages in a row and just 1 (one!) percent have more than two miscarriages consecutively. Trying to conceive after a miscarriage is such a common experience that there's even a special term for the resulting children: rainbow babies. These little miracles are proof that if you can weather the torrential thunderstorm, you just might find your proverbial pot of gold.

My very own rainbow baby inspired me to write this book, because while the road to motherhood can be littered with potholes, the journey is so, so worth it.

When pregnant with a "rainbow baby," it is perfectly natural to feel guilt and fear about the past mixed in with excitement for the future. Honor your emotions instead of burying them. You are not alone.

ENDNOTE: THE FINAL PUSH

Whew! If you're reading this, you're almost done with this book, and maybe with your pregnancy, too. Whether your pregnancy is fraught with every single symptom in this book or none at all, remember that every pregnant body is **DIFFERENT**, and every pregnant woman is **BEAUTIFUL!**

DON'T BELIEVE ME?
TURN THE PAGE TO SEE FOR YOURSELF!

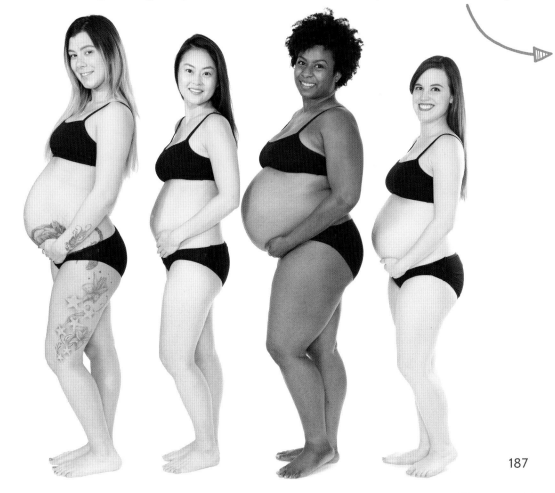

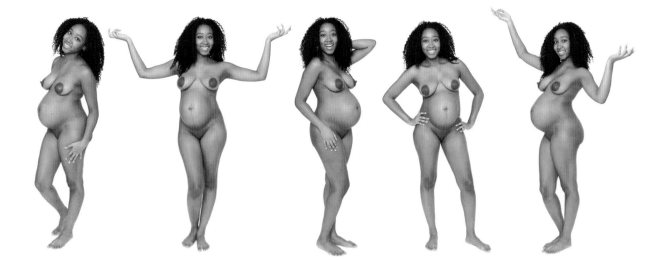

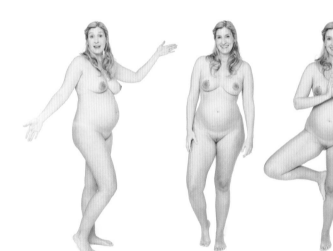

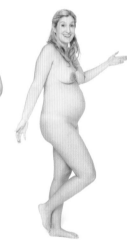

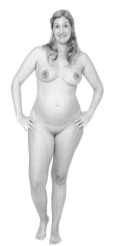

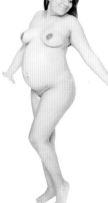

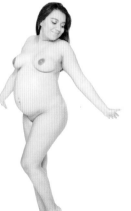

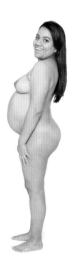

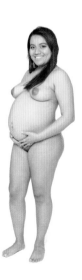

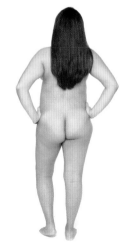

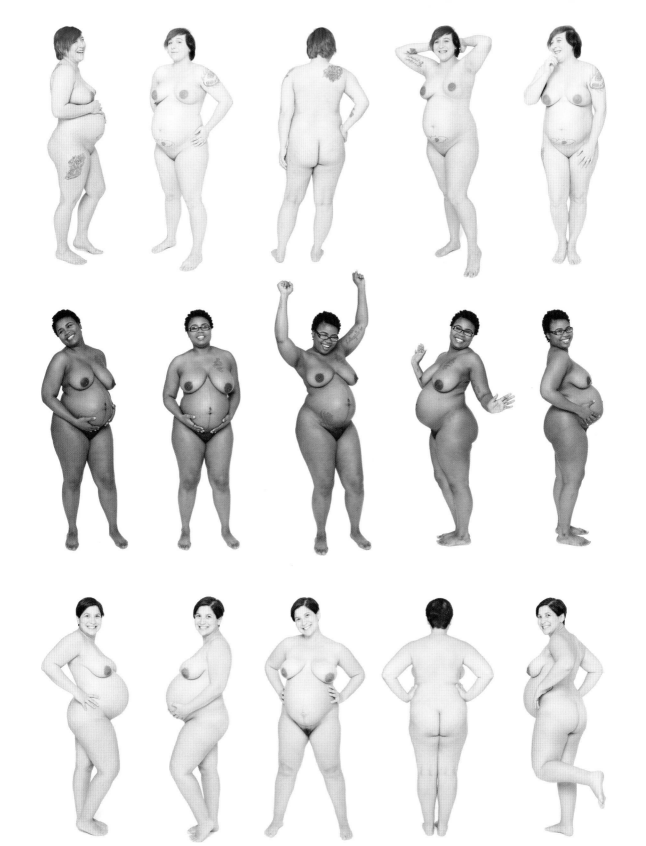

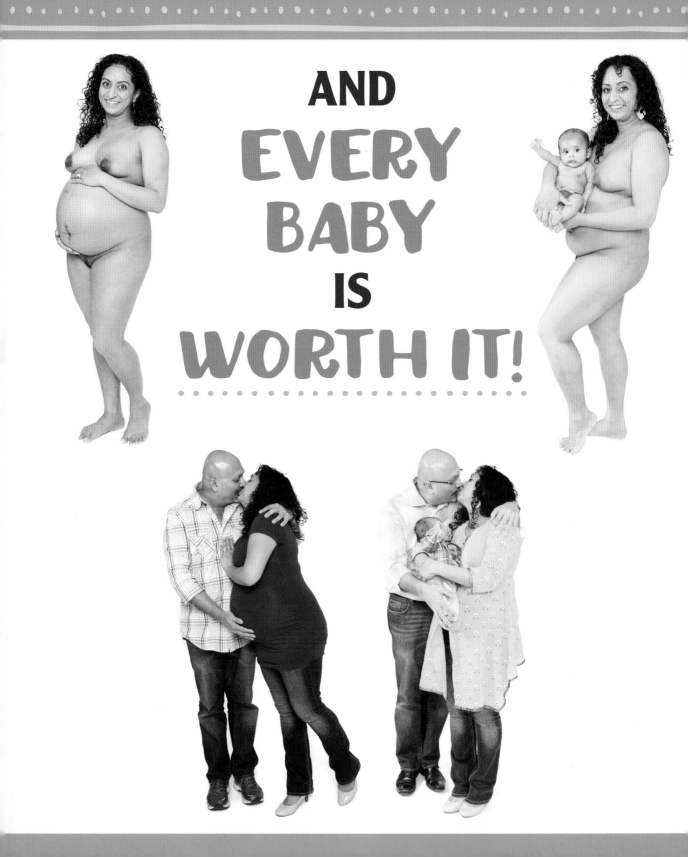

AND EVERY BABY IS WORTH IT!

RESOURCES

Here are some excellent resources to give you even more information about and help with some of the issues mentioned in this book, including phone numbers for free and confidential hotlines.

General Help
All-Options Pregnancy Resource Center
www.all-options.org
888-493-0092

Gestational Diabetes
American Diabetes Association
www.diabetes.org/diabetes-basics
/gestational

Violence & Abuse
The National Domestic Violence Hotline
www.thehotline.org/is-this-abuse
/pregnancy-abuse
1-800-799-SAFE
1-800-787-3224 (TTY)

Domestic Shelters
www.domesticshelters.org

National Child Abuse Hotline
www.childhelp.org
1-800-4-A-CHILD

Financial, Nutrition, & Living Assistance
Government Benefits
(specific to your state)
www.benefits.gov

Child Support & Childcare Help
Administration for Children & Families
www.acf.hhs.gov

Workplace Discrimination
National Women's Law Center
www.nwlc.org/legal-assistance
202-588-5180

While the resources listed are nationwide, many organizations and agencies provide help for millions of local mothers in specific states, regions, and cities. Your medical professional should be able to guide you in the direction of legitimate help if you ask.

Don't get scammed! Unfortunately there are many scammers who prey on vulnerable individuals, taking personal information and even payment in exchange for services and help that never come. Never pay an "admin fee" or any other monetary amount, no matter how small, as that is a big red flag. Stick with organizations that are either official nonprofits, affiliated with a church or other reputable program, or groups that have an excellent reputation around town.

Suicide Prevention
National Suicide Prevention Lifeline
1-800-273-8255

Bed Rest Help
Keep 'Em Cookin
www.keepemcookin.com

Sidelines
www.sidelines.org

Single Mothers
Single Mothers By Choice
www.singlemothersbychoice.org

Loss & Bereavement
March of Dimes
www.marchofdimes.com
1-800-367-6630

Unspoken Grief
http://unspokengrief.com/

CJ First Candle
http://cjfirstcandle.org
1-800-221-7437

Depression
Postpartum Support International
www.postpartum.net
1-800-944-4PPD

Postpartum Dads
Postpartum Men
www.PostpartumMen.com

Mental Health Issues
Mental Health Services Administration
www.samhsa.gov
1-800-662-4357

FYI ABOUT DOCTORS

Midwife? OB? NP? *OMG!*

Because this book is about pregnancy, which is highly medicalized in America, I've written a lot about seeing "the doctor" and talking to him or her about any issue or concern you might have. Some of you may prefer to mentally substitute *doctor* with a doula, nurse practitioner, midwife, OB-GYN, or whomever you decide to put your trust in for the next few months.

> **Remember that the Internet is no substitute for a credentialed health professional, so while Google may be your first stop for advice, it should never be your last.**

When You Don't Trust Your Doctor (or Your Doctor Doesn't Trust You)

You have a right to a medical team that is available, warm, and responsive to your needs. Trust your growing gut. If you do not feel heard or respected, do not be afraid to seek a second opinion or to switch to a different practice. Keep looking until you find the right doctor or health professional for you, even if it's mere weeks before your due date. Many excellent doctors unofficially specialize in last-minute acceptances of patients who flee their previous doctors because of dissatisfaction. You deserve a doctor who respects you and sees you as a mother-to-be and not just Patient 154 of the day.

If at any point during your prenatal care your chosen health professional tells you to plan on going to the emergency room when it's time to give birth, find someone else if at all possible. This is often a warning sign as to the level of interest in your overall well-being. You are entitled to someone who wants to be there for the big event.

Other Doctors You Need In Your Life

Your calendar may be filled with pregnancy-related medical appointments, but don't forget to schedule routine-maintenance visits that may have nothing at all to do with your pregnancy. You only have one body, and as you've seen in this book, there are many ways that pregnancy can take a toll on your health for years after baby is born. Keeping up with your dentist, eye doctor, physical therapist, dermatologist, talk therapist, or other specialists for issues you might have (or develop) is key to staying on top of any temporary or long-term health concerns before they become more problematic.

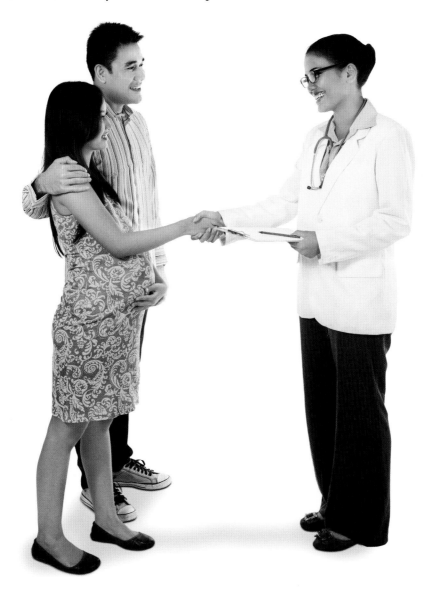

ACKNOWLEDGMENTS

Countless people deserve tremendous praise for helping me birth all of my babies—human and literary! Specifically, however, I would love to shout out my darling agent and friend, Rachel Ekstrom Courage, for being the best book doula an author could ask for; book designer extraordinaire Casey Hooper (caseyhooperdesign.com) for generously bringing my vision to life whilst bravely baking a baby herself; the marvelous Jen Weis, Sylvan Creekmore, and the entire team at St. Martin's Press for believing in this book from the very beginning; phenomenal photographer Brynne Zaniboni (brynnezaniboni.com), whose joyous spirit radiates through her brilliant work; incredible Evelyn Battaglia for cleaning everything up; Dr. Kamilah Dixon and Dr. Sherry A. Ross (drsherry.com) for their eagle-eyed review of everything; Caitlyn Becker and Carla Miskawi for being my right-hand ladies at all the shoots; all the wonderful moms who dared to bare it all both in writing and in photographs; and my hubby Rupak, my kids August and Baby Nancy, my mommy Amanda, my brother Sammy, my wonderful in-laws Sunita and Jahar, along with Devi, Guchi, Ishaan, Rishab, and all other members of my wonderful family. Finally, tremendous thanks to my dear readers and fans, many of whom have followed me from puberty to pregnancy and whom I love with all my heart. Always know that you are not alone, and that we are all in this together!

CREDITS

INDEX

sores, in mouth, 115
spider veins, 16
spotting, 58–59, 157. *See also* bleeding, during
    pregnancy
STDs. *See* sexually transmitted diseases
steroids, 20, 21
stillbirth, 185
stirrup style, 158
stockings, compression, 16
stones, tonsil, 112–14
strawberry kisses, 17
strep infection, 23
stress, 18, 72, 173–80
    fatigue-related, 140
    hormones, 172
    increased, 115
    insomnia and, 149
stress incontinence, 52–54
stretch marks, 11–12
stretching, 6
striae gravidarum, 11. *See also* stretch marks
stroke, 78
subungual keratosis, 97
sugaring, 35
suicide, 179
    prevention, 193
sunscreen, 15
support
    child, 192
    hose, 2
    mental health, 182, 193
    network, 162, 164–65, 183
support groups, 175
    online, 182
sweating, 17–18, 138
swelling, 1, 4–6
    in extremities, 3
    nasal, 80
    normal, 2
    with other symptoms, 3
    reduction of, 2
    sudden increases in, 3
    uneven, 3
sympathetic pregnancy, 155
symphysis pubis, 68

tailbone, 68
tape, kinetic, 67
taste, alteration in, 131
tattoos, 12

tazarotene (Tazorac), 14
teeth, 103–15, 118
    loose, 116
    painful, 116–17
temporomandibular disorders (TMD), 118
temporomandibular joint disorder (TMJ), 118
tension headaches, 72
testosterone, 176
tetracycline, 14
therapy, 154, 165, 175, 195
    couples, 152
thirst, unquenchable, 137
throat, 103–18
thrush
    oral, 112
    vaginal, 56
thyroid, 29, 30
tinnitus, 91, 92
TMD. *See* temporomandibular disorders
TMJ. *See* temporomandibular joint disorder
toenails, ingrown, 98–99
tongue, 111
tonsil stones, 112–13, 114
tonsilloliths, 112
touching, nonsexual, 160
transition to parenthood (TTP), 152
transverse grooving, 98
trauma, during pregnancy, 183
tretinoin (Retin-A), 14
trichomoniasis, 56
TTP. *See* transition to parenthood
tumors
    birthmarklike, 17
    breast, 45
    granuloma, 114
Tylenol. *See* acetaminophen
type 2 diabetes, 138

umbilical cord, 13
umbilical hernia, 13
    postpartum, 67
umbilicus, 13
unplanned pregnancy, 179
Unspoken Grief, 193
urethra, 48
urinary incontinence, 52
urinary tract infections (UTIs), 54, 56, 57
urine
    characteristics of, 54
    output, 4

ABOUT THE AUTHOR

Bestselling author and television host Nancy Redd is a GLAAD Award nominee for Outstanding Digital Journalism, an NAACP Image Award nominee, a Mom's Choice Award winner, and a winner of a National Parenting Publications Award.

She is married to her college sweetheart, actor and writer Rupak Ginn. They have two children, Baby Nancy and August. Nancy is a sought-after speaker and thought leader who utilizes her numerous ups and downs (both literally and figuratively) to effectively champion body acceptance for women of all shapes, sizes, and life stages.

Two weeks after graduating from Harvard with an honors degree in women's studies, Nancy won the title of Miss Virginia and competed in the Miss America Pageant, where she won the swimsuit competition and made the top ten. This experience would become the impetus for her two nonfiction award-winning books *Body Drama* and *Diet Drama*. *Pregnancy, OMG!* is her third book. To contact Nancy, visit www.nancyredd.com.

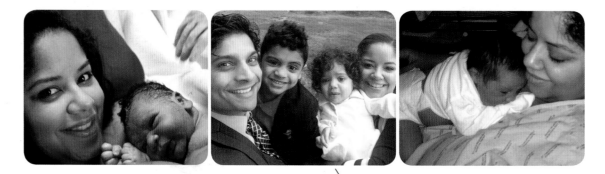

"Smile" does not mean frown, Baby Nancy!